Marilyn Gough

A CARE-GIVER'S GUIDE
Practical solutions for coping with aging parents or a chronically ill partner or relative

Jill Watt

Self-Counsel Press
(*a division of*)
International Self-Counsel Press Ltd.

Copyright © 1986, 1994 by Jill Watt

All rights reserved.

No part of this book may be reproduced or transmitted in any form by any means — graphic, electronic, or mechanical — without permission in writing from the publisher, except by a reviewer who may quote brief passages in a review.

Printed in Canada

First edition: April, 1986
Second edition: March, 1994

Canadian Cataloguing in Publication Data

Watt, Jill, 1931-
   A caregiver's guide

(Self-counsel psychology series)
First ed. published as: Taking care.
ISBN 0-88908-773-3

   1. Caregivers. 2. Aged — Care. 3. Handicapped — Care.
4. Chronically ill — Care. 5. Aged — Family relationships.
6. Handicapped — Family relationships. 7. Chronically ill — Family relationships. I. Title. II. Title: Taking care. III. Series

HV697.W38 1994   649.8   C94-910188-5

Cover photography by Terry Guscott, ATN Visuals, Vancouver, B.C.

Self-Counsel Press
(*a division of*)
International Self-Counsel Press Ltd.

1481 Charlotte Road
North Vancouver,
British Columbia V7J 1H1

1704 N. State Street
Bellingham, Washington
98225

CONTENTS

	INTRODUCTION	vii
1	DECIDING TO BECOME A CARE-GIVER	1
2	ATTITUDES	6
	a. What "they" say	7
	b. Becoming a care-giver: Evaluating your own attitudes	8
	c. Your attitude toward others	10
	d. Your attitude toward the care-receiver	12
3	LIVING ARRANGEMENTS	14
	a. Living together	14
	b. Care facilities	15
	c. Visiting the care-receiver in a care facility	18
	d. Finances	25
	e. Records and important information	26
	f. Promises	26
	g. For the care-receiver: Moving	28
4	HELPING YOURSELF	33
	a. Time management	33
	1. Calendars	33
	2. Lists	34
	3. Telephone messages	36
	4. Where does your time go?	36
	b. Care-receiver's abilities and problems	37
	c. Give others a chance to help	37
	d. Community help	46
	1. Information services	46
	2. In-home services	51
	3. Mutual support groups	52
	e. Start your own collection of resource materials	53

f.	Referral circuit blues	53
g.	Your own medical needs	54
	1. Patient rights: what can we expect?	54
	2. What are our responsibilities?	55
h.	How to choose your doctor	56
i.	Making decisions	58
j.	Words	58
k.	Reviewing your own situation	59
l.	Expert advice on how to cope	60
m.	Bowing out	67

5 PROVIDING BETTER CARE — 70

a.	Eyes	71
b.	Feet	71
c.	Teeth and dentures	72
	1. Toothaches	72
	2. Plaque	73
	3. Mouth troubles	73
	4. Give teeth care	74
	5. Dentures take care	75
	6. Care for partials	75
	7. Food for teeth	76
	8. Eating and dentures	77
d.	Ears and hearing aids	77
	1. How the system works	77
	2. Causes of hearing loss	78
	3. Signs of difficulty	78
	4. Buying a hearing aid	80
	5. The way to start	80
	6. Tips on care	81
	7. Questions and good answers	81
	8. Quick checks	83
e.	Medication	83
f.	Health insurance	84

    g. Create a mini-biography 85
6 PROBLEM AREAS 88
    a. Trust 88
    b. Slight gradual changes 89
    c. Time 89
    d. Job hindrances 90
    e. Recognition 91
    f. Waiting 92
    g. The sweet care-receiver 92
    h. Repetitious chatter and interruptions 94
    i. The unreasonable care-receiver 94
    j. Selfishness 95
    k. Losses and anticipatory grief 95
    l. Terminal illness — a life-threatening disorder 97
    m. Indicators requiring immediate assessment 97
    n. Loss of enthusiasm 98
    o. Loneliness 100
    p. Burial/cremation plans and the will 101
        1. Burial/cremation plans 101
        2. The will 105

APPENDIXES

1 Helpful publications 113
2 Health organizations 116
3 Responses to "relatives caring for relatives" questionnaire 133
4 Dealing with grief 138
5 AIDS/HIV — what to do as a care-giver 140
6 Cognitively impaired and head injury 142

WORKSHEETS

#1	The situation at a glance	5
#2	Analyzing your feelings	16
#3	Assessing the care-receiver's financial affairs	27
#4	Activity assessment checklist	38
#5	Care-giver's daily activities	44
#6	Care-receiver's daily activities	45
#7	Care-receiver's abilities sheet	47
#8	Help sheet	48
#9	Reviewing the situation	61
#10	The professional/community worker's review	63
#11	Outline for mini-biography	87
#12	Burial plans	106

SAMPLES

#1	Care facility information sheet	19
#2	Cover letter to care facility	24
#3	Things-to-do list	35
#4	Directives list	111

INTRODUCTION

This book is for people who are already care-givers or those thinking about taking care of a relative. Care-giving covers a wide range of situations and includes arranging care for a relative as well as caring for the person in your own home.

No matter what you do for the care-receiver, your own physical and mental health must come first. This book helps answer questions you should be asking on coping, but are probably too embarrassed, afraid, or guilty to ask. You must live your own life at the same time that you are arranging the affairs of the care-receiver.

Care-givers frequently feel they can't change their minds once they have made an offer or a decision to care for a relative. This book shows you that you can change your mind and not feel guilty.

If you can read only part of this book, read the first four chapters. Of course, the rest of the book has useful information, but the first chapters give you the basic tools to survive. A positive attitude while you manage both big and little crises combined with health and stamina will sustain you in situations that would otherwise seem totally unbearable.

Many care-givers find it difficult to look at the basic facts of their care-giving. Feelings and emotions tend to invade nearly every aspect of thought and activity. For this reason I have included a variety of ways to overview most types of care-giving arrangements — diagrams, charts, forms, and thumbnail sketches of real care-givers. Of special interest to many of you will be the time sheets that provide space to indicate the amount of time you spend on the activities that sometimes entirely consume your day in "work" with no "play." You may want to photocopy the forms for your personal use.

1

DECIDING TO BECOME A CARE-GIVER

If you have an elderly parent or infirm relative who requires long-term care, you need to determine how much care that person needs and how you are going to provide it. The first step in taking care of a relative who needs your help is assessing the situation. You may assume that your elderly mother, for example, is completely dependent on you and needs everything done for her. But this may not be so. Because of your emotional involvement with your mother, you may be anticipating needs that do not exist. This is a common reaction.

First, then, get a professional opinion to determine the extent of care needed. A doctor can tell you if your relative is in need of help or if she is just putting on an act to get a little extra attention from you. Consider carefully before you commit yourself to taking someone into your home to live. Your mother's apparent helplessness may be her way of saying, "I'd like you to pay a little more attention to me."

Some family members feel intimidated and don't want to hurt a parent's feelings by saying, "You are not really so sick, you know. You can do things for yourself." This is why a professional opinion is important. You need to find out whether your relative has *needs* or *wants*.

Next, you need to be sure of your own feelings. You may agree to take on the care of a relative because you think the responsibility will only be temporary. But the time can stretch out and the situation continue. Before long you may find you don't have a life of your own anymore.

Either you want to become a care-giver or you don't want to; the feeling is spontaneous. If you feel that you *should* do it, then you don't want to. If you have any reservations at all, look at the situation very carefully. Duty alone is a terrible reason to undertake this kind of responsibility.

As the family care-giver, you are the primary person who arranges care for your relative or spouse, whether the care-receiver lives with you, in his or her own home, or in a care facility. You are the one who is responsible 24 hours a day, 365 days a year, which can be a physical, social, and emotional strain.

But you don't have to go it alone. Friends can help. Take advantage of all the free printed material available in your area. Community workers and agencies can guide you to inexpensive booklets that might also be helpful. It is very important to find out what kinds of help are available in your community. The city health and social service departments are good starting points. For some family care-givers, libraries and community centers may be more convenient. (See chapter 4 for more information on community support.)

The outline below gives examples of some of the many realities that have to be dealt with on a day-to-day basis. It is based on the experiences of a family in which the husband suffered a stroke following heart surgery. The left-hand column lists a few events in the care-receiver's experience. To the right are the corresponding arrangements made by his wife.

THE CARE-RECEIVER'S EXPERIENCES	THE CARE-GIVER'S ARRANGEMENTS
Stays alone for the first time since his stroke.	Travels by plane 3,000 miles to get the children from the grandmother's house, where they have been since their father's stroke six months ago.
Travels with family by plane to their hometown.	Makes plane arrangements for two adults and two children, packs, calls a taxi, and checks out of the hotel.
Walks up and down stairs, but has to remind himself which leg to put first and to lock his knees.	Makes sure she's handy to put out a hand when he loses his balance until he is confident on his own.
Goes for daily treatment to the rehabilitation center.	Arranges the appointments at the rehabilitation center and for daily bus to pick up and deliver him.
Has problems with fatigue and must often rest. Goes for medical examination and blood tests.	Arranges medical examination and lab tests and locates a convenient pharmacy.

THE CARE-RECEIVER'S EXPERIENCES	THE CARE-GIVER'S ARRANGEMENTS
Needs help getting in and out of the bath. Can't walk down the basement stairs because the railing is on the left. Is independently mobile, but the fear of falling is always present.	Removes scatter rugs throughout the house and places an extra table and chair in the bathroom for support. Arranges for a railing to be installed on the right-hand side of the basement stairs.
Begins regular walks in a nearby park.	Accompanies husband on walks. Purchases a supply of cane tips as they wear out quickly with regular use.
Removes sling when shoulder soreness subsides, but this affects his balance and for about a week he finds it difficult to walk.	Observes and encourages her husband as he struggles to perform tasks which would be simple to a healthy person.

How do you know whether you are really coping with the situation? Imagine that you have a double and that he or she just appeared and will take over everything for you. You don't have to tell your double anything because he or she knows exactly what to do for your family and the care-receiver.

What would you do right this minute? Where would you go? Would you have your double take your relative someplace so you could relax in your own familiar surroundings? Would you want to go someplace where you didn't know anyone and where you could be catered to? Would you like breakfast in bed? A quiet house so you could sleep? The freedom to make all the noise you can't make when you are looking after your relative?

Just what would you be doing if you weren't looking after your relative or friend's affairs, visiting him, or making her meals, or doing her laundry, or house-cleaning, or shopping, or going to the doctor's office, etc.?

These imaginings can help you discover what you feel is important that you are not getting at all or not getting often enough.

If you are already a care-giver, the following questionnaire may help to clarify your feelings. If you are curious to know how other care-givers responded to this questionnaire, see Appendix 3 for selected answers to each of the questions.

Relatives Caring for Relatives

1. When you became the care-giver was it because of one of the following reasons — duty; you were the oldest; loyalty; closest in age to relative; ill relative liked you best; you wanted to, had the time, knew what to do — or for any other reason?

2. About how long have you been managing the affairs of your ill relative or friend?

3. What are some of the activities you do that help you to manage the ill relative's household, nursing, financial, and social affairs?

4. What are some of *your* activities that especially help *you* with your own affairs (emotional and physical health, social and educational activities, and financial concerns)?

5. What tasks or activities do other people do for the ill relative that you find especially helpful?

6. What things would you like other people to do to help you?

Care-giving is not easy and care-givers often feel trapped. They tell each other in great detail about their problems, sometimes almost competing to see who is the most overworked and miserable. They may try to make better-organized care-givers feel guilty for wanting time for themselves.

Don't waste time with these people. Seek out people, organizations, friends, and family who can *help* you. Avoid anyone who makes your job harder, makes you feel that what you do is not worthwhile, or makes you feel depressed, disappointed, or drained after being with them. People who are really helping you leave you feeling confident, more assured, and better prepared.

You can use Worksheet #1 to sum up the situation before you make specific decisions about how you are going to provide care for your relative.

WORKSHEET #1
THE SITUATION AT A GLANCE

CARE-GIVER

Name_____

Age_____

CARE-RECEIVER

Name_____

Age_____

Relationship to care-giver:

_____

	Yes	No		Yes	No
Works for wages			Health problems		
Regular outside activities			Financial problems		
Financial problems			Mobility/transportation problems		
Transportation problems			Spouse/partner — lives with		
Spouse/partner — lives with			Dependents		
Dependents					

OTHER ASSISTANCE GIVEN

From:

Person/Agency/Organization   Type   How often

_____

_____

_____

_____

2
ATTITUDES

Just who are family care-givers? You may recognize your own situation among those described below.

Tanis, a part-time office worker and student, is trying to hire a reliable housekeeper/companion for her frequently confused mother.

Mary, 58, is considering retiring early from her job because her brother has cancer and is semi-bedridden.

Martha, 40, lives with her parents to help with transportation and household duties since her mother's breakdown.

Ann, 27, an executive with a large department store, visits her mother nearly every noon hour, travelling several miles to the nursing home.

Bill, Caroline, and their young family invite Bill's mother and father to live with them.

Albert, 72, has nursed his bedridden wife for three years.

Colin and Ethel, who are both teachers and have three small children, help Ethel's father care for his sickly wife.

Betty and Alan, expecting their first child, take in Betty's diabetic mother.

Keith, 30, asks for a transfer from his well-paid, on-the-way-up position to his hometown to be closer to his family after his father has had a heart attack.

George, 46, must arrange for a companion for his father who lives 1,500 miles away.

Bill, 32, phones his mother twice a week to "see how things are."

Fay, 62, spends every Saturday with her parents, taking them shopping for groceries and household supplies.

Anyone, in any situation, may find himself or herself being a care-giver. Responsibilities vary, as does the degree of involvement with the care-receiver.

When you become a care-giver, you will experience a variety of reactions from friends, family, and the care-receiver. As well, your own attitude toward the care-receiver and others may change in light of your new situation. Being prepared for these attitudes is one way to cope with a care-giving experience.

a. WHAT "THEY" SAY

From time to time, relatives, friends, and not-so-good friends express opinions on family care-givers. What they say is not always sympathetic. How often have you heard the following?

"The only things she talks about are caring for her father and what she's seen on TV."

"Her father can do a lot for himself...so why does she wait on him hand and foot?"

"We'll worry about money later."

"She has a lot of trouble getting a sitter for her husband, so don't ask her to come."

"In my opinion the family should look after the parents."

"Can't she get the government to do something for her mother?"

"Imagine sending him to one of *those* places! You'd think his daughter would take him in."

"There is only one proper way to look after your mother."

"Old people shouldn't be treated that way."

"He'd be better off in an institution."

"She doesn't visit much...and after all he's done for her."

"You never get good care in a nursing home."

"She's just after his money."

"She didn't talk to him for years, but now that he's unconscious, she visits every day."

"You should always look after your parents *no matter what...*"

"She's marvelous...no help...she does everything for her mother herself."

"She can't look after him at home...her with arthritis and a bad back!"

These are some of the reactions you can expect when you become a family care-giver.

b. BECOMING A CARE-GIVER: EVALUATING YOUR OWN ATTITUDES

There are three essential ingredients to becoming a successful family care-giver:

(a) You must want to, for whatever reason.

(b) You must be prepared to arrange care for your relative and yet keep your own lifestyle and needs in balance, and not neglect your own health in your concern to promote the health and comfort of your relative.

(c) You must be prepared to plan. This includes making decisions, anticipating the care-receiver's needs and your own, and planning for emergencies. If you lack natural abilities in any of these areas you must be willing to learn.

Your mental and physical health should be good enough that it won't deteriorate with the extra responsibility and activities.

Before you assume the responsibility for an ill or infirm relative, examine the quality of life you and your family have. Should you decide to assume responsibility, plan to continue the quality of your life the way you want it; don't throw away what is important to you because of your ill relative. (Reasonable relatives do not want you to give up your lifestyle, they want merely to share in it.) You have your own routine, social life, financial affairs and health, as do the immediate family members living with you. You also have a certain pattern of relationships with other relatives, your friends, and your fellow workers. Think about all these things before you make any decisions.

When you have made your decision, tell several people or write down what you plan to do and why. In times of emotional stress, or when you are tired or frustrated, or when you've just had a bad day, you can talk to those friends or re-read your objectives. Then you can ask yourself, "Am I doing what I said I'd do? Is it too much for me? Have I changed my mind? Should I give it another try? Do I need to make another plan?"

If what you are doing is not what you outlined in your original plan, you need to reassess the situation. Care-givers tend to be very generous people and often find they have taken on more than they can handle, physically or emotionally. If you find this has happened to you, step back and reconsider your commitments.

Are you resistant to change? Hesitant? You're not the only one. Others are also reluctant to disturb their plans. You may have to ruffle a few feathers — those of the doctor, home-care people, nurses, care-receiver, friends, and family — when you remind them of the conditions you originally agreed to when you first consented to become the care-giver.

One woman stipulated, before she took her father into her home, that she would not give up her job, nurse her father, or spend all her money for his expenses as long as he had an income and a bank account. She was prepared to give up a room in her home and much of her time to prepare meals, do laundry, assist with financial matters and legal affairs, and so on. However, she said that when a crisis occurred such as a heart attack or stroke, others in the family would have to manage the problems surrounding the medical care, medical costs, and transportation to and from the care facilities.

Although this was the original plan, this woman gradually found herself handling most of the things she had said she wouldn't do. She was not firm enough with relatives and the professionals she dealt with; she should have reminded herself that she was assuming more and more tasks that she had not agreed to. She knows now, in retrospect, that she should have had definite times to review her position.

As a care-giver, you must reassess your position at regular intervals. If you have taken on more than you agreed to, want to, or can realistically continue to do without the collapse of your own mental and physical health, social and family life, and financial reserves, you have the right to make changes.

But how do you express your feelings? How can you make changes and still provide good care for your relative? Ask yourself these questions:

(a) Where are you going to go for information and advice?

(b) Are you a care-giver only because you don't know how to say no?

(c) If you were offered assistance, would you still want out?

(d) What changes would you like to see?

Begin by writing down the activities you would like help with or would like someone else to take over entirely.

If you do decide to get help, it could be either hired or volunteer, whichever best suits your situation. You could ask other people to perform tasks for you occasionally, when needed or wanted; or regularly, every day, once a week or once a month. You might, for example, ask someone to handle all the necessary transportation, wash all the dishes, or be responsible for telephoning other relatives to keep in touch.

Once you have clarified your feelings and thoughts, you can take practical steps toward improving your situation.

c. YOUR ATTITUDE TOWARD OTHERS

Care-givers usually don't know what to expect of others and they are often quite unprepared for the realities of care-giving. As the family care-giver, you will likely expect certain things of others. For example, you will expect that the health professionals that become involved will look after your relative properly; will coordinate all of your relative's activities (medical, social service, physiotherapy, occupational therapy, accommodation in a care facility); will consider your own feelings; and will give you advice and information, talk about probabilities, and help you make contingency plans when necessary.

On the other hand, you probably won't expect much from other family members, although you may think a lot about what they *could* do if they wanted to. From the care-receiver you will expect that he or she will try to help himself or herself as much as possible and will be considerate and cooperative.

When expectations are not met, you may feel disappointment, dissatisfaction, and sometimes distrust.

For our purposes, consider "expectations" to be those things you think someone will do or say and what you guess, expect, or assume will happen. Expectations also include those things you have been led to believe will happen — from your experiences, family upbringing, education, printed matter, or from the media.

In this regard, I caution you to beware of the "word-fact." John Kenneth Galbraith coined this expression to describe what happens when people begin to believe in something just because it is talked about positively and often. For example, if you hear many positive reports about an innovative project being done at a local hospital, you could jump to the conclusion that the project will be commonplace in all hospitals in two or three years...maybe even tomorrow.

Expectations are not always realized. One care-giver who kept a journal during her husband's illness had this to say about her assessment of the nursing care her husband received: "My comments on the nursing service concerned those things that either failed to live up to my expectations or else exceeded them. I expected my husband to receive certain care and it was only when he did not get it or received more care that I commented on the fact. Similarly, as next-of-kin I expected to be treated in a certain manner. Only when I was not did I write about the incident."

When expectations are not met, a mini-crisis can result. Your reactions to these crises depend on how often you've had to adjust to other unmet expectations in care-giving. You may be rude, or yell, or talk, or be silent, or cry. You may feel that you must "do" something, or you may be angry or feel distrustful or betrayed or confused or guilty. You may nag, or accuse and blame, or complain, or refuse to listen. You may feel you've lost face, or feel inferior, or "know" you are incompetent, stupid, and a failure. You may talk to yourself, saying things like, "No, not yet, not another problem; I'm not ready," and "When will it end?"

Here are some examples of unmet expectations. Try to think of ways that these disappointments could have been avoided.

WHAT HAPPENED	HOW THE CARE-GIVER FELT
A 68-year-old terminal cancer patient who had been chided by the doctor for not getting enough sleep was asked by the nurse to stay awake and let her know when the IV needed to be changed.	The family thought that the hospital nurses did these things for a patient who needed rest.
A 72-year-old father, in the hospital because of a stroke, developed severe bedsores and a rash.	His family thought that such things "didn't happen these days."
A terminally ill patient and her relatives were told by the doctor that "there is nothing more that can be done."	The family felt disbelief and dismay.
A patient and his family were told by the doctor, "You have to expect a little discomfort as you get older."	The family expected that the patient's ailments would be attended to in some fashion, to make him feel better.

The family of a stroke patient was only allowed to visit during visiting hours: 2:00–4:00 p.m. and 6:00–8:00 p.m.	Since stroke patients are often their best in the mornings, the family expected to visit before their relative tired.
The care-giver was not given lists of agencies that might be able to help if she began to feel overwhelmed and helpless.	She felt that "they" don't really care.
A daughter drove her father to the hospital to visit her mother every day for five months.	The daughter began to resent the intrusion into her day, and then felt guilty for feeling that way.

d. YOUR ATTITUDE TOWARD THE CARE-RECEIVER

Remember that someone who is ill has definite ideas on how he or she wants to be treated. You should respect those desires *if they are reasonable*. It is not reasonable to spend every waking minute with the care-receiver just because that's what he or she wants or demands. On the other hand, the care-receiver may wish to be left alone most of the time, particularly if he or she doesn't feel well. For example, don't hover around the hospital room if the care-receiver would prefer you not to. This will only drain you of needed physical and emotional energies.

Care-receivers frequently say, "When I am well..." or, "When I am better..." They may not believe they have a chronic problem, but instead think their difficulties will go away if they rest more, stay in bed, stay indoors, stay away from excitement, eat differently, and so on. It is very difficult to look after a care-receiver who refuses to acknowledge a chronic disorder, especially over a long period of time.

Care-givers also often fail to accept a relative's chronic condition. Care-givers need assistance from others to help them recognize that everything *won't* return to the way it used to be. Crises do occur from time to time in a chronic situation; when a crisis is over, the chronic disorder will still be there.

Those who are not coping with a problem will tend to continually complain, which can make you feel impatient and resentful. When you have had enough of the tirade on, for example, the disorder that your mother has had for six years, say so, and end the conversation: "Mother, I don't want to talk about that anymore. I came over to invite you to supper tomorrow. Will you come? The boys are bringing home some college friends."

Find a way to *express* your feelings and attitudes about the care-receiver. If you feel frustrated, tell a friend, doctor, or neighbor. Verbalize your feelings and regularly assess your attitudes to determine if a change is needed.

3

LIVING ARRANGEMENTS

a. LIVING TOGETHER

Deciding to share your life with an ill or infirm relative will affect your independence and privacy. There are positive and negative aspects to this arrangement for both parties, and you should carefully consider all the problems before the care-receiver moves in with you or you with him or her.

This is not the time to think positively. Think of all the negative points and how they will affect your day-to-day life, not only for a few days or weeks but for years. The care-receiver will not grow up and move away like a child; as time passes he or she may become more dependent. You may begin to feel that the care-receiver is usurping your life, controlling your activities, and making your life miserable.

Don't wait until after the move to consider any possible problems. Find solutions to all negative aspects before any move is made. And look at the positive aspects realistically in light of the greatest length of time that your doctor believes your relative may live.

You may, for instance, be contemplating having your mother live with you until your spouse retires in seven years. After that, your sister plans to take your mother. But in seven years your sister may have remarried or died or become very ill herself.

You should make several contingency plans. Other arrangements will have to be made at some point if you are unprepared to look after your mother when she becomes bedridden, or confused, or incontinent, or has no bowel control, or continues to fight with the children, or your spouse can't stand it anymore. All these potential problems must be faced honestly.

There are also pros and cons to living together from the relative's point of view. If, for example, your father is now living on his own, he will feel the loss of his privacy and independence if he moves in with your family. Whatever the age of the care-receiver, get him or her to read section **g.** of this chapter. If the care-receiver is determined to live independently, this section explains the considerations he or she must make and outlines the options available.

Consider the following factors before you decide to bring an ill or infirm relative into your home:

(a) Your management abilities — arranging and organizing your relative's care and your own home life

(b) Your planning — thinking ahead and planning for emergencies and their effect on those close to you

(c) Your time

(d) Your effective communication — talking with doctors, the rest of the family, your friends, and those of the care-receiver

(e) Your awareness of your own aging (Special points to consider are attitude, personality, energy, activity, mobility, sight, hearing, and finances both now and 10 or 20 years from now.)

(f) Your priorities (What activities will you give up? Some things, nothing, a lot? Be prepared to give up some of the time you used to spend on your own activities. Since another person is present, you will also lose time alone to think, reflect, plan, or just be quiet. It may become difficult for you to accept impromptu invitations from your friends or to go out for an evening on the spur of the moment. And since you have another person to consider, you won't always be able to do things *your* way.)

Worksheet #2 on the following page was designed to help you analyze your feelings and those of your relative as you consider whether or not you should live together.

If your care-receiver is already in your home, use Worksheet #2 to reassess your feelings. Jot down your main concerns and feelings in the appropriate areas. Look at them, talk about them and think about whether you feel the same now as you did before. What are the differences? What caused your feelings to change? What can you do about it? Do you want to do anything about it?

b. CARE FACILITIES

There may come a time when, in the best interests of you and your relative, you decide to find an appropriate care facility.

You may be limited in your choice, but start by talking to the care-receiver's doctor and your own (if you have a different doctor), the community nurse, your pastor, your neighbors, and any friends

WORKSHEET #2
ANALYZING YOUR FEELINGS

CARE-GIVER	CARE-RECEIVER
feels GOOD about	
(positive)	(positive)
(negative)	(negative)
feels UNCOMFORTABLE with	

who have relatives in nursing homes. Check the Yellow Pages and call the library to see if they have a list of extended care/seniors' housing facilities in your community. Collect as much information as you can.

At this time, a nursing home may not be the most suitable place for the care-receiver. Other accommodations to consider are shared residences and easy-care apartments. Those under age 60 may not want to be in housing with mostly senior residents. Some seniors don't want to be just with older people; they like to see and hear children too. Talk with both your friends and the care-receiver's; look at brochures from the various facilities, co-operatives, societies, rental and for-purchase apartments and condominiums. This may be all the information you need to select the new residence.

Save yourself time and energy by using a questionnaire to assess the facility. Sample #1 shows a Care Facility Information Sheet. You can use this form or compose your own special list of questions and mail it to three or four care facilities.

Your questionnaire should ask for basic information such as, "Are there open visiting hours?" "Is there a bed available?" "How big is the facility?" "Is there easy parking?" or "Is the facility on a bus route?" Later, when you visit the two or three top possibilities, you can concentrate on the important things that don't easily fit questionnaire forms: atmosphere, comfort, suitability for your relative, friendliness, cleanliness, what the residents are like, and so on.

Send the questionnaires to the care facilities accompanied by a covering letter (see Sample #2) and enclose a self-addressed, stamped envelope. Include your telephone number in the covering letter if you wish and state if you are available during business hours. (Most care facility business offices are open 9:00 a.m.–5:00 p.m. with another number for emergencies after business hours.)

After the questionnaires have been returned, pick those points that are of special concern to your care-receiver and ask detailed questions of the care facility administrators over the phone. Don't waste your time going to visit the place before you have taken this step.

Some of the types of questions you might consider asking are —

- How soon do you expect to have a private or semi-private room available?
- Can my father have his own remote-control TV in his room?
- Is there someone on all shifts who can irrigate and/or change a bladder catheter?

- When, exactly, are the visiting hours?

Then make appointments to visit the two or three places you are seriously considering. It is true that making an appointment allows the people who own the facility to prepare for your visit and show the facility at its best, but it also means they will be prepared to spend time with you, answer your questions, and give you a tour of the place. On the other hand, if you visit the facility unannounced, you take the chance of not being able to talk to the people who can give you answers, but you will be able to gauge the facility for atmosphere, cleanliness, safety features, size, and convenience.

c. VISITING THE CARE-RECEIVER IN A CARE FACILITY

In most care facilities, you will meet at the bedside. Although your relative may prefer meeting you in the lounge or on the sun deck, you will most frequently be visiting your spouse or relative in his or her room.

"Visit" may sometimes be an inappropriate word as it suggests friendliness, sharing, talking, companionship, and laughter. Your care-receiver may be in a coma, or confused, or watch you and appear to listen but never talk.

In a situation where the care-receiver does not contribute to the conversation, visiting is simply being present. Some care-givers stay for long periods — they take reading material (if the light is good) or sewing or letters to write. Others may sit for a few minutes and go home or else go to the lounge and return later to "see" the care-receiver and allow him or her to see the visitor.

As the care-giver, you are observing how your relative is being looked after. You are looking for things you might want to attend to, such as purchasing more toilet articles, doing some laundry, or passing on messages to your relative, the staff or the resident in the next room.

The care-receiver who communicates all or much of the time should be consulted on the quality and type of visits he or she prefers. You may not be able or want to satisfy an unreasonable care-receiver, but most residents' and patients' wishes can be fulfilled easily. Some care-receivers will want frequent visits, others will want many visitors and still others will ask for specific family members and special friends.

The care facility may have visiting hours, a few a day. These hours can be changed, should your circumstances and the best interests of

SAMPLE #1
CARE FACILITY INFORMATION SHEET

Care Facility Information Sheet

Type of service provided: _____
(For example, Personal Care, Intermediate, Extended, Acute, etc.)

Number of patient/resident beds in the facility: _____

Name of care facility: _____

Address: _____

Phone number: day _____ night _____

Hours business office is open: _____

1. ADMISSION AND FEES

- Are there eligibility requirements for admission such as age, sex, religions affiliation, language, or other?
- Do you have space available now?
- Do you have a waiting list?
- How are patients/residents admitted?
    —By doctor referral?
    —By another care facility or social worker referral?
    —By self?
    —By family?
- Does the facility require a contract?
- What are the charges per month? Per day?
- Are monthly statements and bills issued?
- What is the refund policy?
- Is a recent medical examination of patient/resident required?
- May the patient/resident retain his or her own doctor?

SAMPLE #1 — Continued

- What notice is required when a patient/resident leaves the facility?
- To whom and when do patients/residents give notice in advance for a short stay away from the facility (e.g., afternoon outing or weekend with relatives?)
- Visiting hours? Unrestricted? Or limited to what hours?
    - —Are children permitted?
    - —Are pets permitted?

2. STAFF
    - What are the shift hours/times?
    - Who is in charge (title) during the day? During the night?
    - Is there a registered or graduate nurse on duty 24 hours a day?
    - Who should be contacted (title) on each shift to obtain information on patient's/resident's condition?
    - List of services; please indicate if each is included in monthly room charge:
        - —Assistance with eating
        - —Assistance with shaving
        - —Assistance with oral hygiene
        - —Assistance with washing hair
        - —Assistance with reading and writing letters
        - —Wheelchairs
        - —Physiotherapy
        - —Occupational therapy
        - —Oxygen
        - —Incontinence aids
        - —Other
    - What arrangements does the facility have to provide these services:
        - —Laboratory
        - —Hairdressers
        - —Barbers

SAMPLE #1 — Continued

- —Podiatrists
- —Dentists
- —Other

- Do staff working directly with patients/residents speak clearly in English ( ) Other ( )
  (if *Other*, please give details)

- How are staff addressed (e.g., title, surname?)

- How are patients/residents addressed (e.g. surname, first name)?

- Is a doctor on call/available 24 hours a day when patient's/resident's own doctor cannot be reached?

3. PATIENT/RESIDENT ROOMS

- What furniture is in the patient's/resident's room besides the bed?

- Are personal furniture and belongings permitted?

- Is own TV permitted? Is there cablevision? Is earphone required? Is own radio permitted? Is reception good in the facility?

- Is shelf provided for books, etc.? Is a corkboard provided for greeting cards, etc.?

- What are the dimensions of the room? Cupboard?

- Can a patient/resident in bed see out the window?

- Where are the emergency buzzers/bells located?

- If patient does not have a private toilet and bath, where are the ones he or she is to use?

- What lighting does the room have and where is it?

- Is private phone permitted?

- Where are the public telephones and can they be reached from a wheelchair?

- Where is smoking permitted?

SAMPLE #1 — Continued

- Are the colors of walls, doors, etc., such that they help patients/residents to orient themselves?
- Corridors: Are there handrails? Are they lit at night? Are they easily negotiable for wheelchairs?
- Does the facility have a lounge? Dining room? TV room? Smoking room?
- Is there an elevator to all floors?
- How often do you have instruction and fire drills for staff and patients/residents?
- Does the facility have automatic fire sprinklers? Smoke detection devices?

4. MEALS AND OTHER SERVICES
   - When are meals normally served?

      —May patients/residents have them at other times?
      —Does facility prepare special diets? Is there an extra cost?
      —At what time of day are the patients/residents provided with their menu choice sheets?
      —How many different weekly menus are there? (Please enclose sample.)
      —Are snacks available?
      —Are visitors allowed for meals/snacks? (If yes, what are the charges?)
      —Do patients/residents have access to kitchen facilities?

   - Is laundry included in the room charge?

      —How much of the patient's/resident's laundry does the facility do?
      —What are the charges for more laundry than that normally done?
      —Do patients/residents have access to any laundry facilities?

SAMPLE #1 — Continued

- Does the facility have a library for patient/resident and visitor use?
- Where is the nearest public library?
- Does the bookmobile visit the facility?
- Are there chapel services?

5. ACTIVITY PROGRAMS
    - Briefly outline the activity programs, indicating which are planned and implemented by facility staff, facility volunteers, community organizations, etc.
    - The activity coordinator is normally available in the facility during what hours?
    - Is transportation provided for patients? Cost?
    - Are sidewalks and streets near facility suitable for invalid walks and wheelchair use?
    - Can facility be reached easily by bus?

6. OTHER
    - Use this space to note any other pertinent information.

Name of person giving information:
Title:_____

Date:_____

SAMPLE #2
COVER LETTER TO CARE FACILITY

                                        Jane Smith
                                        1234 Any Street
                                        Anytown, Anwhere
                                        (Telephone: 555-6543)

Best Care Haven
4321 Home Street
Anytown, Anywhere

Sir/Madam:

    Enclosed is a questionnaire requesting information about your care facility. I am looking for a suitable facility for my mother.

    The information you send will assist me in selecting the appropriate accommodation for my mother.

    Thank you for your time.

                                          Sincerely,

                                          Jane Smith

your care-receiver warrant it. Either you or the care-receiver's doctor can discuss the matter with the administrator of the care facility.

Fixed facility visiting hours are not in the best interests of residents and patients. Visitors, residents (or patients) and staff should, in cooperation with each other, consider the quality and quantity of socializing appropriate for each individual as well as considering the time and feelings of the care-providers (family and professionals).

d. FINANCES

You should make financial arrangements with the care-receiver before you enter into any agreement. If you are already involved in caring for your relative, tackle the points in this finance section now if you haven't already. Many care-receivers do not have a realistic idea of the cost of living today, particularly if they have been ill or infirm for some time.

If your relative is seriously ill, irrational, or dying, bankers suggest that you look into the following:

(a) The possibility of borrowing money to cover the period of illness and/or lifetime

(b) Whether any money should be transferred from the sick person's account to your own (with his or her consent) (A lawyer should be consulted in this matter.)

(c) Write a financial statement of the care-receiver's affairs

Nursing homes, hospitals, home-care program staff, and others who provide service will all expect to be paid. It is important that you know what your relative can afford and consider how much of your own money, if any, you can contribute.

Worksheet #3 will help you assess your relative's financial resources. You can then discuss what he or she desires in accommodation, goods, and services and explain what, if anything, you are prepared to give financially.

Care-givers usually fail to keep track of out-of-pocket expenses like time spent, gas, wear and tear on the car, food and lodging, etc. The cost of caring for your relative should be recorded — even though you may never collect. (Bear in mind that the care-receiver is unlikely to leave something in the will for you. Your relative may not consider what you are doing as "helping," but rather as your duty.)

A record of expenses lets others know what your assistance is costing you, especially should they begin to think that you are gaining financially from the caring position. Such a record is also handy should you decide, temporarily or permanently, to allow someone else to take over the primary care-giving role. It shows in print that you have helped, that you have managed the care-receiver's affairs for a period of time, and what it cost you in out-of-pocket expenses. This also helps the new care-giver to gauge costs, time, and energy and compare it with what he or she had anticipated.

e. RECORDS AND IMPORTANT INFORMATION

Well-organized people keep all their records together, even if they are not in any kind of order. You will need to keep track of many records and pieces of information for the care-receiver if you are living together, or even if you take on the responsibility of finding alternative living arrangements.

To start, keep everything in an envelope. Then increase the size of the envelope as needed. Later, you will need a shoe box, and perhaps, eventually, some space in a filing cabinet.

As you gather more records, you can organize them by category (e.g., hospital, house, car, etc.). The main thing to remember is to keep everything together. Perhaps you will have boxes within boxes, *but keep them in one place.*

If you are the care-receiver's spouse, you don't need to keep his or her records separate from yours unless you are living apart. For example, you may be at home but your spouse may be in a hospital.

f. PROMISES

Don't promise things. Don't lie. You can be both honest and comforting.

Relatives sometimes say, "Promise me you'll never put me in a home/hospital/away...?" or, "Promise me you'll take me in when I'm old and can't do things anymore?" These pleading requests and, sometimes, demands for you to promise something should not be responded to with, "Of course we'll look after you. Don't be silly thinking we'd put you in a home."

Frequently, a hospital is the *only* place where treatment can be administered. Or, your circumstances may be such, for whatever reason, that you can't reasonably keep your promise. It's better not to make any promises in the first place. Reply in ways that are reassuring. For example, "Mom, we'll look after you — how, I'm not sure, but we'll see that you are given the best we can." Or, "There

WORKSHEET #3
ASSESSING THE CARE-RECEIVER'S FINANCIAL AFFAIRS

INCOME		ASSETS	
Pensions	$_____	Stocks	$_____
Employment income	_____	Bonds	_____
Rental income	_____	Term deposits	_____
Interest and dividends from investments	_____	Real estate	_____
TOTAL	$_____	TOTAL	$_____

HOUSE COSTS		PERSONAL COSTS	
Mortgage	$_____	Food	$_____
Rent	_____	Clothes	
Property tax	_____	—purchase	_____
Insurance	_____	—washing	_____
Hydro, fuel, water	_____	—dry cleaning	_____
Sewer	_____	Income tax — quarterly (March, June, September, December) or annually	_____
Refuse removal	_____		
Building maintenance	_____		
Grounds maintenance	_____		
Appliances	_____	Barber, hairdresser	_____
TOTAL	$_____	Medical/health/dentist	_____
		Telephone	_____
		Cablevision	_____
		Cleaning person	_____
		Grooming purchases —toothpaste, soap, etc.	_____
		Miscellaneous —stationery and postage	_____
		—transportation	_____
		—entertainment	_____
		TOTAL	$_____

isn't room for another adult, Mom, but we'll figure out something when or if the time comes."

Say what you feel. Let the relative know that you care but don't promise things you can't be sure about or may not feel the same way about five, ten, or twenty years from now.

One care-giver refused a transfer to another town with a large increase in salary and increased status in the firm because he and his wife had promised his mother (after Dad died) never to leave her, and she wouldn't move with them even though they wanted to take her.

g. FOR THE CARE-RECEIVER: MOVING

There are pros and cons to living together. If your care-receiver is determined to live independently, get him or her to read this section. Independence can be a boon to health and well-being. There is help for those who want to continue living on their own.

Moving and the independent older person*

If you like where you are living, stay there as long as you can. You have a routine and you are familiar with everything that is around you. If you have some difficulties, a homemaker service, mobile meals service, and nursing services may be your solution. Some service clubs provide transportation for doctor's appointments and outings. If you are happy where you are, try to use all the services in the community.

Many people don't realize that less than 15% of elderly people ever move into institutions. And only 1% ever get so seriously confused that they may be called senile. Most of us — at least 85% of us — live on our own. We do our little bit to help others less fortunate than ourselves and we enjoy life. Although we may wonder at these "new-fangled things" and ways of the younger folk, we get along just fine.

If you do have to move, take with you some of the things you value most. And what do you value? Well, imagine that you have been picked up and deposited somewhere that gives you shelter, food, clothing, and company. These are four of your basic needs. Then the boss gives you permission to send for a few things (your wants). Ask yourself, "What will I miss most?" Next, ask, "What will I send for?" Some of you will

---
*This section was prepared by Jill Watt for the Consumer's Association of Canada (B.C. Branch). Reprinted with permission.

answer husband, cat, my own room, garden, telephone, my collection of books, easy chair, or remote control TV.

The secret of a good adjustment to a new residence is to take with you what you value. Take as many things "that you can't get along without" as possible and you will adjust more easily to a new home. You may have to sell, store, or give away some of your belongings, but you don't have to do it right away. You will have time later when you are more settled to decide what you can do without.

Some of you may welcome moving to some other place but you don't know how to go about it. Perhaps you don't like where you are staying, or you have come to the point where it is very difficult taking out the garbage, getting the groceries, or preparing meals.

If you have these troubles, perhaps you shouldn't wait for a relative or friend to suggest that you look for another place to live.

Talk to a social worker or to someone at the health unit in your area about finding accommodation to fit your requirements. Your needs have changed — you now need a little bit of assistance to move.

Usually when you move, it means going into something less than what you now have. Perhaps you can stay in your own home if you are subsidized and use some community homecare services. If subsidies are not available or the homecare medical services are not possible, you will have to accept a move.

Many studies have been done to see what effect moving has on people. The experts suggest that adjusting to a new location is easier if you choose accommodation in the same area or a similar type of area. It seems that it is not so stressful if you keep some of the familiar surroundings and social activities of the community that you have lived in for some time. If you do have to move out of your area, try to pick another that is similar. Don't pick one that is way out in the country if you are used to city living. If you are a country resident, don't choose a high-rise. The noise, the hustle and bustle and the crowds might be a little frightening to someone who is not used to it. If you are accustomed to peace and quiet, look for that type of atmosphere.

You'll never find exactly what you want — be prepared to compromise a little bit.

Any move is going to disturb you. This happens to everybody. It doesn't matter whether you are a senior citizen or not.

When you move, get a lot of help. Don't let yourself get tired. Let your friends help — they want to. If you don't want to ask them outright for assistance that probably they would give gladly, invite them over so they can see what kind of mess you are in. Give them an opportunity to find out what your needs are and allow them to offer to help you.

If you are suddenly hit with a medical disability and are told that you can't stay where you are because you need too much assistance, tell everyone who is helping you to relocate what type of place you would like. If you want a private room, be emphatic about it and put your name down on a list. There is a shortage of single rooms and private bathrooms. Many operators of residences and administrators of hospitals rationalize this by saying, "But old people like living together," "Seniors like sharing," and "The elderly don't like to be alone." All those things may be true under certain conditions, but most of us do like a room of our own even if we like the company of friends and relatives too. And a bathroom of our own is another thing that most of us are accustomed to.

If you are in one of the following situations you may need someone outside to help you and to talk to your relatives:

(a) You've made up your mind to move and where you'd like to go, but your relatives and friends have chosen another place for you.

(b) Your relatives have asked you to stay with them but you don't want to (the reason doesn't matter). You haven't decided where you do want to live but you don't want to live with them.

(c) You are already staying with relatives and you don't want to stay there anymore.

(d) Your relatives all want you to stay with them for awhile and you don't feel up to shuttling back and forth between them all. You'd like to have a home base.

(e) You are in a place of your own or you are living with relatives and the relatives think that you should go into a mental institution. You don't want to go, nor do you feel that you should have to.

(f) You are with relatives and you don't want to be there and they don't want you to be there either, but no one is doing anything about looking for another place for you, so you all argue all the time.

(g) You want to live with your daughter or son because you can't cope on your own any longer and you believe that children should take care of aged parents. But yours don't want to.

(h) You are in a place of your own and you can't bear to go anywhere else. You want to stay where you are. "I am going to stay," you say, "they will have to take me out bodily." Well, that is exactly what is going to happen. If you cannot stay where you are for financial or medical reasons and you don't have another place to go to, then someone is going to come along and pluck you up and put you in a residence or hospital whether you like it or not.

In the chart below, accommodation options are listed in order of increasing dependency on others and decreasing personal privacy. As one descends the list of options it is common and usual to be sleeping in a room with one or more people and sharing a bathroom. Many of you will want to look at the options in both lists because of your special circumstances.

Money will buy you more independence and privacy, as you can have a private room in a residence, care facility or hospital — if it is available.

ACCOMMODATION OPTIONS

Financially handicapped	Medically handicapped
• Small apartment house, or condominium	• Your residence with incoming help
• Share residence with someone	• Your residence with live-in help
• In your home — relatives live in	• Your residence with a relative living in to help
• In-law suite in relative's home	• Relatives' residence with their help
• Senior citizen housing	• Relatives' residence with their help and incoming help
• Live with relatives in their home	• Rest home (personal care facility)
• Guest house or rent home	• Intermediate care facilities or private hospital
	• Extended care facilities or acute care hospital

Outside help can come from many sources: your doctor, your local health unit, your friend, your minister or priest, the public health nurse, the social worker at the health unit. Other than the friend, all the persons listed are professionals who are used to talking with people, especially relatives, and doing counselling and referral work. They would be glad to help you decide where you want to live and to talk to your relatives for you.

Think of your independence and privacy *before* you move or you might lose them.

4

HELPING YOURSELF

a. TIME MANAGEMENT

Care-givers tend to be very generous when giving of themselves and their time. Consequently, they frequently overextend themselves to the point of physical and mental exhaustion. When this happens the care-receiver is bound to suffer also. (See Dr. Nicholls' comments near the end of this chapter.)

As a care-giver, your time will be wasted in the relationship unless you know your priorities and where your time goes. The information that follows is designed to help you see where you have been spending your time and where you need to make changes. If you find the care-receiver taking an increasing amount of your time, you may have to consider alternative arrangements.

Generally, the stay-at-home family care-giver is lucky to get one evening out of the house a week. Even the simple decision to visit, window-shop, or see a movie requires extra energy, thinking, planning, and arranging. Here are some ways to help you manage your time and allow you to "get away from it all" periodically.

1. Calendars

A calendar is an absolute necessity. Appointments are easy to remember when you have them marked down on an easy-to-read, large-format calendar. Some people use a calendar instead of making lists, but I suggest that beginner care-givers use both.

Mark down the things you must do and the things the care-receiver must do so you can see the whole picture at a glance. When there are changes in plans (as often happens) you merely adjust your daily schedule. If you have a commitment at a time when a health professional wants to set up an appointment, you'll know right away and can suggest alternate times.

A purse or wallet-sized calendar that duplicates the larger one at home is also helpful. It provides you with the information about upcoming activities and allows you to make additional plans. It also shows those you are in contact with that you are efficient and realistic. Taking on more than you can handle in a day is poor management and often results in fatigue and irritability. Conserving your energy for priority activities is most important to you and your care-receiver.

Events and items recorded on your calendar will include doctor's appointments, home nurse visits, banking, homemaker days, barber or hairdresser appointments, visits with friends, outings, holidays, birthdays, and anniversaries, etc.

2. Lists

Almost all competent, well-organized people use lists of some kind. Time-management experts recommend using lists for organizing your day.

You can make lists for yourself or others for the purpose of delegating family chores and clarifying instructions. Lists are visual print-outs of what you do and plan to do. A list can help you show others what you do and where they can help, should they offer.

A "to do" list is the beginning of planning — it separates your regular routine from occasional activities. With this list and a calendar of commitments and appointments, you can arrange most caregiving activities around the framework of your planned activities.

Always involve the care-receiver in scheduling his or her activities and encourage him or her to plan each day up to a few weeks or a month ahead. Planning for today, tomorrow, and the next few weeks is not unreasonable as long as what is being planned is relatively feasible.

There are many different ideas for list-making but all share the same basic concept of being a checklist or reminder of things which must be done. Sample #3 shows one useful design.

If you put your shopping list at the lower corner of the page you can tear it off without affecting the other items.

Don't attempt to list items in order and don't put down routine chores. If you change your bed linen every Friday, don't put it on your list. However, if you are making a list to leave with a helper, you'll have to remember to list all chores, including the ones you perform by habit.

SAMPLE #3
THINGS-TO-DO LIST

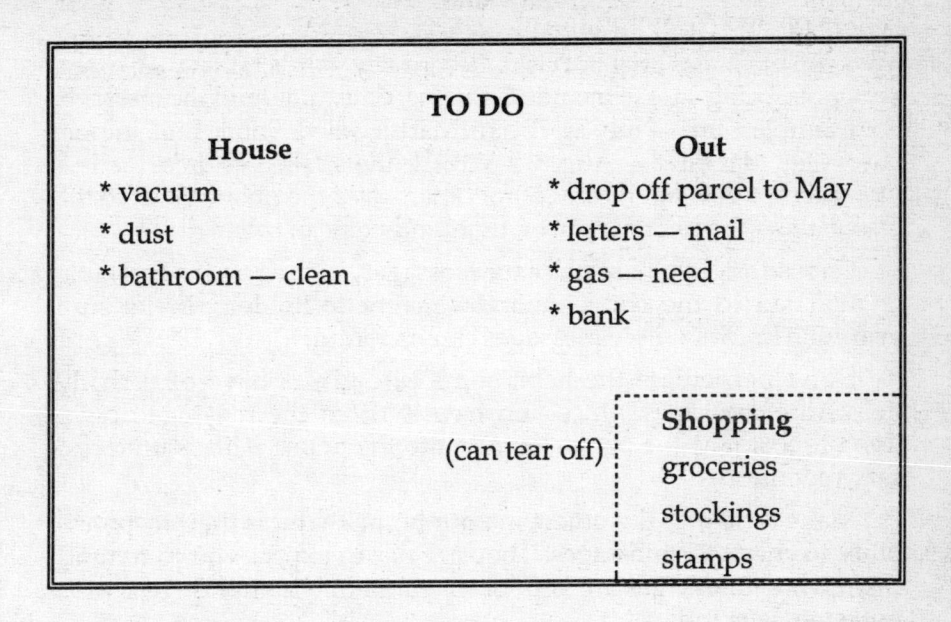

```
                          TO DO
         House                         Out
    * vacuum                     * drop off parcel to May
    * dust                       * letters — mail
    * bathroom — clean           * gas — need
                                 * bank

                                   Shopping
                 (can tear off)    groceries
                                   stockings
                                   stamps
```

Try not to put any task on the list that you don't plan to complete within a couple of days. You'll find it discouraging if you can't accomplish the items listed.

If you do find that some items are carried over onto your list for several weeks, try to think of an alternative way to accomplish the task. One care-giver wrote on her list, "Weed the garden" for four weeks; finally she changed it to "Phone for a gardener."

An item that continues to be carried over should tell you something. You may need to forget about it, pay someone to do it, or do it less often. Perhaps it has become routine and shouldn't be on the list anyway. Maybe you should drop the item as being something that might be nice to do "if you have the time."

One care-giver put down "write letter to mother" so many times without following up that she eventually wrote "phone mother during cheap rates and chat." She felt relieved because making that decision removed the guilty feeling of having failed to write a letter of two or three pages. She gave herself permission to spend the money on phone calls once in a while on the grounds that letters took more time and phoning gave both her and her mother more satisfaction.

3. Telephone messages

Consistency saves time and a regular place for messages prevents confusion and disappointment.

Keep messages brief but clear. Record key words rather than entire sentences, being sure to include the name, date, time, and the message. For example: "Jim — July 24, 10 a.m. Martin called. Phone him. Important." Or, "Margaret — Aug. 3, 2 p.m. Cleaners called — dress ready." Don't accept detailed messages for others over the phone. Stick to the essentials — the phone number, time, and name of caller.

Choose a convenient place for messages, such as on the hall table or attached to the fridge door by magnetic holders. Make sure everyone knows where messages can be found.

Don't perpetuate the habit some care-givers have of verbally delivering messages. Once you have written the message down, don't repeat it as the person comes into the house. This is unnecessary repetition.

Make it clear to the others in your home that it is their responsibility to check for messages. They are not to expect you to remind them where messages are kept or to tell them whether there is or is not a message today.

A telephone answering machine, if you can afford it, is another efficient way of recording messages for members of your household.

Now, absolutely none of this is appropriate for the care-receiver who has a vision, hearing, or comprehension problem. The personal delivery method must always be used until you find out how much sight, hearing, or comprehension loss your relative has and what communication system is best suited to his or her abilities.

4. Where does your time go?

Assessing where you are and, from time to time, assessing your care-receiver's condition and your own activities is crucial to maintaining a good relationship. Worksheets #4, #5, and #6 are included to help you assess both what you do and what your care-receiver can do.

First Worksheet #4 will help you to see the overall picture. How much time do you spend on yourself and on your own family? How much time do your care-giving activities require?

Then, every couple of months, review your situation and evaluate how it has changed. Record the date of your review beside any comments you have. This exercise will help you to look objectively at your situation. Do you have a healthy balance between personal and care-giving activities? Or is care-giving gradually usurping most of your time and energy?

You may also want to use the daily activity sheets to monitor your time and the care-receiver's time on a daily basis (see Worksheets #5 and #6).

b. CARE-RECEIVER'S ABILITIES AND PROBLEMS

Worksheet #7, which assesses the care-receiver's abilities, is valuable for several reasons. If you are deciding whether to become the care-giver, it will enable you to see what assistance your relative or spouse will need every day. If you know what must be done daily, you can figure out how much time it will take and when you must give that time. Knowing this is vital before deciding to become the care-giver. You must have time for yourself.

If you are already the care-giver, this sheet can be used for other purposes:

- You can fill it out for yourself at regular intervals to see how the care-receiver's condition is changing
- On the basis of these changes, you can decide whether you should continue as the care-giver
- A care-receiver's abilities sheet provides needed information about the care-receiver's physical abilities to anyone you may need to call in to help out — temporarily in an emergency or on a regular basis.

c. GIVE OTHERS A CHANCE TO HELP

When people ask what they can do to help, be specific. Make a list of tasks that other people can help with, and when someone offers assistance, show him or her the list. If you give people a choice of tasks, they are more likely to respond positively.

Anyone who offers help will want a brief explanation of the job to be done. On your task list, include a few words describing the job. Generalizations are enough: list details of jobs only if absolutely essential.

If a friend or family member offers to help and then shows no interest in any task that is on your list, don't give up. Ask that person what they had in mind when they offered to help. You may find that they can help out in a useful way that you had not considered.

WORKSHEET #4
ACTIVITY ASSESSMENT CHECKLIST

Where your time goes	Activities you do	Amount of time	Activities you arrange to be done	Amount of time to arrange	Comments
Making bank deposits					
Record-keeping					
Paying bills, writing letters and checks					
Mail - receiving, sorting, reading and dealing with same					
Social letter-writing - friends and family					
Paid work in or outside of house					
Decision-making and planning menus, purchases, decorating, maintenance of accommodation and furnishings					
Attending school - day, night, occasionally					
Supervising work of others					
Supervision of own children					
Sleep					

WORKSHEET #4 — Continued

Where your time goes	Activities you do	Amount of time	Activities you arrange to be done	Amount of time to arrange	Comments
Daily bathing and personal grooming					
Eating					
Reading magazines, newspapers, books, etc.					
Radio - listening					
TV - watching					
Exercise					
Visiting friends					
Phone visits to and from friends and relatives					
Attendance at your club, society, organization, community center, etc.					
Sports - active in					
Sports - watch					
Show, movie (film), concert, pub, tavern, cocktail, disco, bingo, etc.					
Dinner out					

WORKSHEET #4 — Continued

Where your time goes	Activities you do	Amount of time	Activities you arrange to be done	Amount of time to arrange	Comments
Hobby - garden, stamp collecting, needlework, etc.					
Interests - studying Egyptology or philosophy, etc.					
Driving car - enjoying					
Volunteer work					
Community and church work					
Vacation - planning and taking					
Taking family members to appointments, meetings, etc.					
Chauffeuring family members to their activities					
Helping family members with their activities such as homework, projects, social engagements, sports, leisure pursuits, etc.					
Walking dog					

WORKSHEET #4 — Continued

Where your time goes	Activities you do	Amount of time	Activities you arrange to be done	Amount of time to arrange	Comments
Feeding animals					
To barber					
To hairdresser					
To doctor					
To dentist					
Purchasing groceries, sundries, clothing, etc.					
Putting away groceries and purchases					
Clothing and linens - making, sorting, mending, repairing					
Dry cleaning					
Shoe repair					
Laundry and ironing - collecting, sorting, washing, ironing, putting away					
Meal preparation - regular, snacks, serving food, setting table, breakfast, lunch, dinner					

WORKSHEET #4 — Continued

Where your time goes	Activities you do	Amount of time	Activities you arrange to be done	Amount of time to arrange	Comments
Clearing table and doing dishes (loading and unloading dishwasher)					
Baking for freezer					
Canning and preserving foods					
Tidying up house					
Making beds					
Housecleaning - regular mopping, dusting, vacuuming					
Floors - wash and wax					
Eaves and tile drainage checked and cleared					
Appliance repair and maintenance					
Furnishing — repair and refurbishing, upholstering, redecoration					
Clean and defrost fridge					
Freezer defrosting, cleaning and inventory					
Clean oven					

WORKSHEET #4 — Continued

Where your time goes	Activities you do	Amount of time	Activities you arrange to be done	Amount of time to arrange	Comments
Windows — washing					
Caring for house plants					
Care of car — tuneup, wash					
Snow removal					
Garden and yard — lawn mowing, sweeping, raking, tidying, edging, pruning, planting flower beds, weeding, car port, garage, entrances, patio					
Furnace filter change and maintenance					
Fireplace cleaning and flue maintenance					

WORKSHEET #5
CARE-GIVER'S DAILY ACTIVITIES

	Activities	Comments
12:01 a.m. to 6:00 a.m.		
6:00 a.m.		
7:00 a.m.		
8:00 a.m.		
9:00 a.m.		
10:00 a.m.		
11:00 a.m.		
12:00 noon		
1:00 p.m.		
2:00 p.m.		
3:00 p.m.		
4:00 p.m.		
5:00 p.m.		
6:00 p.m.		
7:00 p.m.		
8:00 p.m.		
9:00 p.m.		
10:00 p.m.		
11:00 p.m.		
12:00 midnight		

WORKSHEET #6
CARE-RECEIVER'S DAILY ACTIVITIES

	Activities	Comments
12:01 a.m. to 6:00 a.m.		
6:00 a.m.		
7:00 a.m.		
8:00 a.m.		
9:00 a.m.		
10:00 a.m.		
11:00 a.m.		
12:00 noon		
1:00 p.m.		
2:00 p.m.		
3:00 p.m.		
4:00 p.m.		
5:00 p.m.		
6:00 p.m.		
7:00 p.m.		
8:00 p.m.		
9:00 p.m.		
10:00 p.m.		
11:00 p.m.		
12:00 midnight		

Use the Help Sheet shown in Worksheet #8 for anyone who offers a helping hand.

d. COMMUNITY HELP*

There are services to help care-givers in most communities, whatever the age or needs of the family member or loved one you are helping. There are also agencies that offer support to you as a care-giver. Specific organizations are not listed because these services vary in their titles and programs from community to community. Services may be offered by voluntary associations and societies, government, or private (for-profit) organizations. Often services and organizations overlap; however, there is often excellent coordination and cooperation between some agencies and government departments.

Unfortunately, it is not always easy to find the agency best suited to your care-receiver's needs. Be persistent and creative; link with all the services and benefits available. Keep track of all the organizations you call and the person you speak to. You may need to contact the organization again for more information or to pass on knowledge you have gained.

Start with your care-receiver's doctor and with your local public health office. (In the United States, those involved in eldercare can contact the regional Area Agency on Aging Office.) Ask for the names and phone numbers of the specific services and groups you want, as well as the name of a contact person. Other care-givers are also a valuable resource. Ask them which organizations they have found helpful and effective.

1. Information services

First on your list of people to contact should be the reference librarian in the Health and Sciences Division at your local library. Ask for a local information directory that includes agencies serving care-givers. Get the phone number of the group that publishes the directory in case there are new listings or changes since publication. Many libraries maintain a list of local support groups. These may be specific to an illness or a health condition or a general care-giver support group.

Other sources of general information about local resources include the following:

- Social work staff of community and children's hospitals

---

*By Shelagh Armour-Godbolt, editor of "Continuing Care Resources Newsletter," Armour Health Associates Ltd.

WORKSHEET #7
CARE-RECEIVER'S ABILITIES SHEET

Is the care-receiver able to —

    Feed self? _____ Require assistance? _____
    Bathe self? _____ Require assistance? _____
    Dress self? _____ Require assistance? _____
    Walk? _____ Require assistance? _____
    Use mechanical aids? List: (e.g., cane, walker)
    _____ _____

See well enough to move about safely? _____

Read printed material? _____

Smell? (e.g., smell smoke) _____

Hear well? _____

Control bladder and bowel? _____

    If not, does he or she maintain own cleanliness? _____

Communicate well? _____

Understand well? _____

Wander away? _____

Disturb others? _____

Act destructively or aggressively? _____

Take own medication? _____

    Require assistance? _____

    How often? _____

Amount of time out of bed each day? _____

How often out of the house and how long?

In your opinion, who and what type of person should look after this care-receiver?

What type of accommodation do you think would be best for this care-receiver?

WORKSHEET #8
HELP SHEET

Care-receiver's personal requirements	Will do	Can help with
Banking: Letters: writing and reading • personal • business Transportation: to and from dentist, doctor, barber, hairdresser Supper: preparation and serving Food: purchase of Personal grooming items: purchase of Bathroom linen: • wash once a week • change twice a week and when needed Clothes: • purchase • assist with washing and ironing (once a week and when necessary) • dry cleaning — take to Bed linen: • wash once a week and when necessary Telephone calls: • assist with making • answer and take messages Assist with: • walking • climbing and descending stairs • rising if fallen (People with bad backs may not be prepared to do this.)		

WORKSHEET #8 — Continued

Care-receiver's house requirements	Will do	Can help with
Top floor: • vacuuming and dusting, etc. as required • cleaning as required • stairs — vacuuming once a week and as required Main floor: • dusting once a week • vacuuming once a week • dishes — wash once a day • tidying as necessary • mop bathroom floor once a day and as necessary • mop spots on kitchen floor as necessary • oven — clean every two months or when necessary • fridge — clean every three months • indoor plants — water as necessary • hall — spot clean and vacuum as necessary • windows — inside, clean every three months • windows — outside, clean every six months • garbage — put out for collection • recreation room — vacuum, dust, and clean once a week Other areas: • veranda/patio — tidy and spot clean once a week • yard — keep garden litter-free • plants — plant or remove in season • weeds — remove as necessary		

WORKSHEET #8 — Continued

Care-receiver's house requirements	Will do	Can help
• place and put away garden furniture as required • prepare soil — cultivation and fertilizing, etc. • edging beds • edging lawn • tidying up • pruning Garage: tidy as necessary Basement: • food locker — check once a week for spoiled, smelly foods • utility area — keep reasonably clean and tidy • workshop area — keep reasonably tidy • stairs — vacuum, dust, and clean once a week		

- Local seniors' center
- Peer counselling programs
- Neighborhood Houses
- YWCA/YWHA
- Veteran's organizations
- Family Services agencies

Your employer may also offer an employee assistance program or counselling. Check the Yellow Pages for services (try "Social Services Organizations" and "Homemaker" or "Domestic Help" listings.)

Contact the regional headquarters of your faith group to see what information they have about community and government services or what local congregations offer on a volunteer basis. Check with regional representatives of retirement organizations such as the American Association of Retired Persons and the Canadian Association of Retired Persons. Contact the retirees' group at the care-receiver's former workplace. Even if the care-receiver is not yet of "retirement age," the group may have helpful resource information for someone forced to leave work because of health problems.

The variety of services available, once you make the right connection, is great. They can range from financial support to subsidized home renovations or special transportation to cope with disabilities, from low-cost legal advice to counselling for either the care-giver or the care-receiver.

2. In-home services

In-home services can include meal services, help with daily household tasks or maintenance, and visiting health professionals (doctor, nurse, rehabilitation therapist, community nutritionist, etc.). The local Arthritis Society or organization for the blind can be helpful resources for adapted equipment, as can the Occupational Therapists Association. Volunteer telephone reassurance calls and visitor programs are often available. Check with the local Red Cross office about short-term equipment loans (e.g., a wheelchair, bath seat, or walking frame).

The care-receiver may benefit from community services such as supervised outings, day centers and programs, paid or volunteer companion services, community meal programs, and recreation programs for people coping with special needs, either physical or mental. Often special needs recreation programs are offered in the evening at local schools, community education offices, or parks and recreation departments. Churches and temples offer weekly or monthly activity days for young people with disabilities, to give care-givers a day off.

If you feel you can't risk leaving the care-receiver alone, ask your local public health unit about subsidized or volunteer companion services. There are personal alert systems that the care-receiver can use if an emergency arises when he or she is alone. Companion services may be privately run or provided on a non-profit basis through a local hospital or nursing home.

Talk to your physician or to the local public health unit about the availability of short-term spaces in nursing or convalescent homes or group homes for persons with mental challenges. Sometimes a short-term space can be booked in advance when you know a special event will take you away from home for a few days or a few weeks. Alternately, some communities offer 24-hour and live-in home companion or help services. These can be purchased for a weekend off or longer. Some services may be subsidized: be sure to ask.

Information about long-term or permanent supported or supervised accommodation is also available from the many sources suggested earlier. Even though this may not be what you have in mind now, ask about the best sources for this information. It is best to find out early; often there are waiting lists.

3. **Mutual support groups**

There are associations that help care-givers who are coping with a loved one who has a serious illness or medical condition. Multiple sclerosis, Parkinson's arthritis, strokes, ALS, Huntington's Disease, AIDS, head injury, etc., all have local mutual support groups. These may be for the affected person or for family members and friends. There are also groups for people who are parenting children or youth with special needs. The pediatric social worker in your local hospital or public health unit or your school counselor or school nurse should be able to link you with "parents of special needs" groups.

Many mutual support organizations have excellent national newsletters at reasonable subscription prices. You can subscribe even if you do not wish to become more involved with the organization. This is another way to make sure you know about the latest research, resources, or coping tips. Most important, contact with mutual support groups gives you the comfort of knowing that "I am not alone."

Keep an organized record of the agencies you contact and keep track of services that you think you might use. This will help you reduce your stress as a care-giver. When you share the care-giving with family or friends, keep track of who does what and when. This way no one's effort is duplicated. As your care-receiver ages or as health needs change, more services may become available. By keeping track of everything you've learned, you can offer knowledge and comfort to other care-givers.

e. **START YOUR OWN COLLECTION OF RESOURCE MATERIALS**

Take advantage of all the free printed matter available in your community. There are also inexpensive booklets and books that agencies and community workers can tell you about.

Sometimes the amount of information you receive can be overwhelming. To help you assess and deal with information, printed or verbal, approach new information by asking these questions:

- (a) Can I use this information to be more effective in my work? In my life?
- (b) How can I use this information?
- (c) In how many ways?
- (d) How soon? When?

You may be eligible to obtain free or low-cost help in caring for your relative in your home. If your relative lives alone, he or she may also qualify for assistance of various kinds.

f. **REFERRAL CIRCUIT BLUES**

The family care-giver is frequently a referral victim — passed on to one agency after another and from one department of a service to another. The "referral circuit blues" is no laughing matter when it happens to you.

The easiest referral is one contacted by someone else for you. To avoid as much hassle as possible from bureaucracies, delegate. Give your problem of getting help or information to someone else. This may appear sneaky, but if you think about it you'll realize that you don't have time to run from one office to another or make numerous phone calls. This is one instance where a friend or relative can be a tremendous help.

When you are in an office and told that Department A, for example, can't help you, ask who might and would they call to confirm. If they won't call, don't stop there. Get them to give you the agency's address and phone number and the name of someone to talk to (a name helps when you first go to an office or make an appointment even if you never see or meet that person). The employee may say, "Well, I don't have the name of the place and address handy, but if you look in the phone book you'll find it." You should reply, "I'll wait — I have time." Yes, you do have time to wait for something like this because if they don't have it at their fingertips how are you going to find it quickly? Wait. If you continue to sit there, they'll find the information for you.

Now, you are doing this for two reasons. First, if you can't find the information in the phone book at home, you are back on the referral circuit a second, third (or more) time around. The other reason is that if a department can't help you, they should at least be able to supply a decent referral — the name of the organization that can help you, and the department, address, phone number, and name of a person to contact.

And do keep a contact list — a box of names and agencies. As you collect names and organizations, hang on to them. You may need them again or a friend might.

g. YOUR OWN MEDICAL NEEDS

As stated earlier, care-givers often over-extend themselves and wear themselves out mentally and physically. One way to help avoid this is to have regular check-ups with your doctor.

You should have a different doctor than your care-receiver. This is contrary to the family practice concept of medicine, but with long-term care you want to preserve your dignity and sanity (and that is what this book is all about). I have come to the conclusion that a different doctor for you and your ill or infirm relative is in the best interest of everyone, unless you are absolutely certain that your doctor sees you and the care-receiver as two people with distinctly different needs.

1. Patient rights: what can we expect?*

Many patient rights are not guaranteed by law. In other words, we don't have the legal right to insist upon them. However, we feel there are fair principles that we, as patients and health care workers,

*Reprinted with the kind permission of SPARC (Social Planning and Review Council of British Columbia). Originally published in 1978.

should operate by. It is our right to *insist* upon competent and courteous health treatment.

We have the right to receive competent and skilled health care provided by an adequate number of staff.

We have the right to considerate and respectful care regardless of lifestyle, income, culture, educational background, or diagnosis.

We have the right to information concerning our medical care and procedures in language which we can easily understand. In such cases where it is not possible to give such information to us directly, the information should be made available to people we appoint to act on our behalf (e.g., family, friends, translators, lawyer, chaplain).

We have the right to know which, if any, of our treatments are experimental and the right to know what alternative treatments exist.

We have the right to participate in decisions involving our health care.

We have the right to refuse any particular treatment or procedure.

We have the right to seek consultation in our health care, to change our physician, as well as the right to be aware of any health care units specializing in our health.

We have the right to know the names and occupations of all health workers involved in our health care.

We have the right to be addressed at all times by the name we prefer.

We have the right to respect and privacy. Our case consultations, examinations, and treatment are confidential and should be conducted discreetly.

We have the right to expect the health care system to act upon our requests.

We have the right to prompt care, especially in emergency situations. The following are examples of priorities for medical treatment: cardiac arrest, unconsciousness, bleeding.

We have the right to a healthy environment within the health care system, e.g., reduced noise levels in hospitals; smoking restricted to designated areas.

2. **What are our responsibilities?**

Whenever there are rights, there are also responsibilities. To improve our health care, we can assist in the following ways:

We are responsible for following a healthy lifestyle in order to minimize health risks.

We are responsible for being honest and direct about everything that relates to us as patients in the health care system. We should tell those who are caring for us exactly how we feel about the things that are happening to us.

We are responsible for understanding our own health problems to our own satisfaction. If we have questions, we should ask our physician and/or other health workers. Understanding our health problem is important for the success of treatment.

We are responsible for telling those treating us whether or not we think we can, and/or want to follow a certain treatment.

We are responsible for telling our physician or health care worker about any changes in our health.

We are responsible for knowing and telling our physician the names of medications and over-the-counter drugs we have been taking, or whether we have stopped or changed medications.

We are responsible for notifying our health care worker (or his or her supervisor) whenever care is unsatisfactory.

We are responsible for knowing the name(s) of the physician(s) treating us.

We are responsible for being considerate of other patients and for respecting their rights to privacy.

We are responsible for notifying our health care worker if we cannot keep a scheduled appointment.

We are responsible for knowing our health history, e.g., allergies, record of treatment in hospital, past operations.

Working together in this manner will ensure continuity and quality of health care.

h. HOW TO CHOOSE YOUR DOCTOR*

Be honest and open in your dealings with your doctor and insist that the doctor is honest with you. If you take his or her advice, then follow it — don't leave out parts. (For example, if the instructions are "lots of fluids and rest," don't drink a lot of tea and then go back to work.)

---

*Reprinted courtesy of the Consumer's Association of Canada (B.C. Branch.)

If you disagree with the doctor, say so. The doctor may not understand your way of life and priorities. There may be another type of treatment.

Do not expect detailed information from the doctor. Have a written list of questions with you when you go to the office. For example, you might ask the following:

- Can you do anything for my problem?
- What is my health problem?
- How long does the cast stay on as I have to tell the office something?
- How long will I be on this medication?
- How much does it cost?
- Is surgery the only solution?

If you and the doctor are not compatible, consider changing to a different one. There are many reasons why you might want to change your doctor — the location of the office; no elevators; the doctor is too slow; religious differences; age; you are moving to another town; the behavior of the receptionist, nurse, or secretary (have you reported rudeness and inappropriate staff behavior to the doctor?); the doctor doesn't listen, doesn't do anything, doesn't understand, is retiring soon, doesn't communicate, is too old-fashioned, or too way-out; or for any other reason.

If you have decided to change doctors, choose a new one before leaving your present doctor.

You could be referred to the new doctor by the doctor you are leaving. Otherwise, find doctors' names by asking family, friends, the public health office, the local association of physicians and surgeons, and your local medical society. Also look in the Yellow Pages under "Physicians."

Consider these points when selecting a doctor: Does the doctor make night calls, homecare calls (house calls), for you only or for the whole family? Does he or she do any surgery? (If so, what type?) Is he or she willing to deal with your stress and tension problem without necessarily prescribing medication? What hospital does he or she work out of? Is he or she in partnership or a member of the clinic or on his or her own? What medical school did he or she attend? How much experience has he or she had? Call the local licensing or regulatory body to see if he or she is registered.

Your next step is to interview the doctor. Spend half an hour with the doctor (possibly at your own expense) to see if you like his or her attitude and answers to your questions. If all goes well, try him or her out the next time you have a problem.

You'll need to transfer your records to the new doctor. Either ask the new doctor to arrange to get your records or phone the former doctor's office to notify him or her of your decision and ask that the records be transferred to the new doctor. (If there is a problem, put the request in writing. Usually the records themselves are considered the property of the doctor who wrote them, but the pertinent information must be given to the new doctor.)

If you are leaving your former doctor because of a complaint, write to him or her saying why you have made the change and send a copy of the letter to the local association of physicians (licensing or regulatory body).

i. MAKING DECISIONS

It's possible that the family, family care-giver, and care-receiver will not like any of the choices when a decision must be made. Worse, the whole family may have varying ideas of what should be done and who should do it.

At times like this, there is a tendency for no decision to be made. Everyone continues to go on worrying and wondering what is going to happen and who is going to do various tasks.

One solution is that you all agree that on a certain day or at a certain time a decision must be made. (See Dr. Nicholls' comments near the end of this chapter.)

j. WORDS

Use appropriate words when discussing care-giving with family, the care-receiver, professionals, and community workers.

For example, if you are shy, nervous, reluctant or in awe, say so, but don't say "fear," "afraid," or "scared." Such words tend to make others back off a little and look at you differently. It is important to you and the care-receiver for you to be explicit in what you say.

Telling the nurse that you are scared or afraid when you are giving the care-receiver treatment is not the same thing as saying that you would like more practice under supervision, that you would like her to show you a technique again, or asking her to watch you because you feel you are clumsier than you should be.

When you ask for help, put your request in simple and direct words that everyone can understand. You will encourage your listeners to respond with the same kinds of words.

Follow this same rule of thumb when discussing your own role with professionals, other relatives, and your friends. To avoid misunderstanding, be specific. Vague words only produce problems. Avoid using words like "busy," "care for," or "do for." Rather, let the people you deal with know a little of exactly what it is you do.

Instead of saying you must "work," say that you must go to your job downtown, organize the charity drive, plan Dad's new diet, organize your garage for the sale on Saturday, or shop for a wheelchair.

Instead of "busy," say that you will be cleaning Mom's house, washing and setting Mom's hair, shopping for groceries — it takes about two hours — or taking Bill to the doctor for his appointment and waiting for him.

If you must turn down an invitation, explain why. For example, say, "Not Tuesday, that's the night we visit John's mother in hospital and catch up on the family news. We take her some of her favorite foods."

Don't be surprised if you find that you're not always on the same vocabulary wavelength as health professionals. Consider, for example, the question, "Has he any complaints?"

The layperson generally uses the word "complaints" to mean criticism of goods or services. Some patients will become defensive when a doctor abruptly asks, "And what are your complaints today?" They reply, "No complaints, but I do have this tightness in my chest. Do you think it is anything I should be worried about?"

When doctors and nurses ask about your complaints they are not asking if you or your care-receiver are dissatisfied or considering a lawsuit by complaining about something. They are asking what is troubling you or what problem you have that they might be able to help alleviate. Doctors consider fatigue a complaint, as well as a rash, a sore shoulder or back, an earache, not being able to see like you used to, and so on.

k. REVIEWING YOUR OWN SITUATION

Worksheet #9 is useful for the long-established family care-giver for periodic quickie review of how she or he is managing. It can also be useful to help the beginning care-giver see the types of things that could be built into cooperative effort of the family care-giver, professionals, and community workers. It is a sort of "temperature-taking" to see how well you are working with the people and resources in your community.

Worksheet #10, the Professional/Community Worker's Review of the Family Care-giver's Situation, has been included here so you can see what some of the people who work with you and your relative may be concerned about. You may also want to give a copy of this form to one of the workers who helps you if you feel that they could be less critical, more helpful, use more words you understand, or be more communicative and understanding of your situation. The form allows professionals to evaluate their communication techniques. The result: more effective care and treatment of the care-receiver. The responsible people who are helping you to be part of the effective care-managing team for your spouse or relative will only expect you to do those tasks that you feel you can handle. Also, they will not suggest more activities without considering your existing schedule, your plans, and your feelings.

1. EXPERT ADVICE ON HOW TO COPE

Dr. Peter Nicholls, a practicing psychiatrist in Vancouver, British Columbia, has ideas and suggestions for those caring for relatives and concerned for their elderly. This is how he answered the following questions.

Q: What if the care-giver is taking care of the relative out of duty alone?

A: We have a kind of bank account of warmth and empathy, but there comes a point when it is exhausted. If you continue to try and give from an exhausted account the result is not a communication of warmth or care or effective functioning. It is irritability, however carefully disguised. The people we work with are immensely sensitive to the covert message of rejection. They are not fooled one minute when your emotional bank account is exhausted.

When the person doing the caring is actually doing it out of duty and not love (or has never liked the individual), that is not a workable situation. It would then be important that you enlist other people who do have a genuine and spontaneous affection for the person to care for your relative.

Nobody owes anybody anything. In fact, the way things are, your emotional and psychological debts are pretty well cleared from moment to moment, but there is that feeling on the part of some people that you owe them.

WORKSHEET #9
REVIEWING THE SITUATION

Date of review _____

1. Were you given adequate description and instruction regarding what you would be doing? Yes_____ No_____
2. Were you given enough background information about your relative? Yes_____ No_____
3. Have you met all the professionals and community workers? Yes_____ No_____
4. Do you report your relative's condition to anyone regularly? Yes_____ No_____
5. Have the professionals/community workers maintained regular contact with you? Yes_____ No_____
6. Do you feel your relative is benefitting from your involvement? Yes_____ No_____
7. Do the professionals/community workers give you detailed instructions about new tasks they would like you to do for your relative? Yes_____ No_____
8. Are you included during evaluations and assessments of your relative? Yes_____ No_____
9. Do you feel you have received adequate training for what you are doing for your relative? Yes_____ No_____
10. Do you feel the professionals/community workers appreciate your contribution? Yes_____ No_____
11. Do you feel your relative appreciates your contribution? Yes_____ No_____
12. How long have you been the main family care-giver? _____
13. What are some of the reasons you became the care-giver?

_____

_____

WORKSHEET #9 — Continued

14. What satisfaction(s) have you had as care-giver?
    _____
    _____

15. What frustrations have you encountered?
    _____
    _____

16. What things do you feel need improvement?
    _____
    _____

17. Do you know where to get additional help in your community?
    _____
    _____

18. Note any other thoughts.

_____   _____
Name of family care-giver   Name of relative being cared for

WORKSHEET #10
THE PROFESSIONAL/COMMUNITY WORKER'S VIEW

Date of review _____

Name of patient/client _____

Name of family care-giver _____

1. Description of the family care-giver's contribution and activities with the patient/client.

   _____
   _____
   _____

2. For what period of time has the family care-giver agreed to undertake this responsibility? _____ weeks _____ months

3. Has the family care-giver received adequate instruction and the information necessary for activities with the patient/client?
   Yes _____ No _____

4. How much time does the family care-giver spend with the patient/client? _____

5. When did the family care-giver last get in touch with you (by phone or in person)? _____

6. How often do you see the family care-giver? _____

7. What things could the family care-giver do that would help you (with the patient/client) that isn't already being done?

   _____
   _____

8. Is the family care-giver maintaining his or her own health (physical and mental)? Yes _____ No _____

9. Are there any ways you could help the family care-giver? What are some of the ways?

   _____
   _____

Name of professional/community worker _____

Q: What if the care-giver feels guilty and/or doesn't feel comfortable dealing with the relative?

A: Anticipatory grief? Guilt? Communication problems? If it interferes with your normal functions such as sleep, appetite, interest in sex, interest in your normal hobbies, your capacity to relate — when you find you are being affected in such a way — one of the first things to do is bring in outside people as resource persons, preferably, but not necessarily, with the care-receiver's approval. The second thing to consider is a discussion with the care-receiver. You may be surprised to hear that he or she feels your sense of guilt or concern is unnecessary, or even a burden. Sometimes people let things go until their relative is mentally incapable or dead, and then they feel they have missed an opportunity.

People too often are giving one another a blank check, and I think that is a strong inducement to developing a hostile, dependent relationship. People are not nearly as fragile as we think they are. When they come into your home or your life in a new way you are entitled to say, "Okay, we are going to look at our new relationship as it develops every so many weeks and we are going to renegotiate our agreement." Review this every few weeks because your relative's condition changes, and so do your feelings.

Q: How can the care-giver cope with looking after a relative every day?

A: Primarily you must look after yourself too. That means being able to move in close at times but also to distance yourself. Having that capacity, in effect to change gears, to work effectively with the distance between yourself and the person you are caring for is a critical issue. When the going gets rough and you feel you are really stretched to the limit and you are trying too hard, you have to be able to back off and take a mental health day or mental health hour for yourself and look after your own interests.

Distancing yourself allows you to put the whole situation into perspective and to recoup your losses — to renew your ties outside the relationship with the ill/infirm person and to add to your emotional bank account. Bring in a second person, a consultant to help you. He need not be someone who is an authority in any sense or a person like a medical specialist. He may be a friend, a neighbor, a priest, or anybody who is more objective and is outside the situation and can give you his views about it.

Everybody must have his own private space within his own head as well as within the geographical space he lives in. Intrusion of another's life into one's own space mustn't be allowed. You have to circumscribe within your own life the area that you need to live effectively. You have to make a decision about that and put up "no trespassing" signs, otherwise you can become emotionally exhausted. Sometimes it's just a matter of putting doors on rooms where there aren't any, both within your own mind and within your house. Sometimes it's a matter of having your mother-in-law live across the street rather than in your own house. Sometimes it is simply a matter of moving across the room. There are a number of different ways of looking at distance. Hearing the same story for the "nth" time you may simply have to hold the phone away from your ear for a period of time to get your feelings under control to be able to deal with that person. If they are living in the same house with you, you may have to move apart for a period of time. You may have to put that person in a hospital over a weekend or for a week or two while you take a vacation from the relationship — you may not even go away. Another way is to put a professional person between yourself and the care-receiver.

If you look after yourself effectively you will be able to look more effectively after the care-receiver. Encouraging optimal functioning on the part of the care-receiver will relieve a lot of the burdens of the care-giver.

Q: What can the care-giver do if the relative is unreasonable?

A: Realize what can be changed and what cannot be changed. I think you have to distinguish between two things: the person who is unreasonable because he is made that way (he is unreasonable about many things in his life and has been for a long time) versus the person who is being unreasonable in this particular situation for a reason. If the person has a certain kind of character problem that is interfering, you shouldn't expect that you will be able to change that. In fact, nobody may be able to. On the other hand, if it's a situational problem, then you can do a multitude of different things to get leverage on the situation. For example, if you take the problem of depression, you often find that people become isolated because of a loss. They experience grief but this is perpetuated because of the consequence of the depression, fatigue, not sleeping well, poor appetite, and so on. They then have less energy to renew ties, to build new ties and move outside of the depressed position they are in, which causes them to be more isolated; and the more isolated they get, the more depressed they get and they get into a vicious circle.

This happens in communication between people, too. Because there is a problem that has not been effectively solved, people are feeling bad about that problem — they may even feel hopeless about it. Because they feel that way, they deal with the problem less effectively than they did before and because they deal with it less effectively, they feel more hopeless about it and so on into a downward spiral.

Look for the point of leverage and you identify the most effective way to deal with the problem. You have to look at the particular relationship itself to find where the point of leverage is, but there are some things that you think of immediately. First — stepping back from it so that you can't get locked into a hard and fast position on the problem. Second — discarding that feeling of hopelessness.

Q: What if the care-giver has trouble making decisions?

A: Procrastination is one of the real problems of the person who is the care-giver — not making a decision but saying, "Oh, wait until tomorrow or next week." So give yourself a period of time in which to make a decision, because decisions are made for you sooner or later if you don't make them yourself. If the decisions are made for you by events or by the people around you, you lose control of the situation. To have some control over your own life you do indeed have to make a decision in a certain period of time. You may as well think about that period of time in advance.

For a small decision, or even for a large one, set a specific time and say, "I'll think about it for so long, perhaps a week. Next Thursday morning the decision has to be made." Be realistic and recognize that a certain portion of the time, maybe 30 or 40% of the time, you are going to make the wrong decision. At least it is your decision and as an adult you can take the responsibility for it. If the decision is made for you, it's very hard to accept the responsibility for the mistake that you made and to change the situation. You tend to blame other people or blame the situation for the mistake. It is adult to take responsibility for yourself. Once you take that responsibility you can feel in control of your life and you can feel good about your successes. As long as there are more successes than failures, the likelihood is that you will feel good about yourself.

Q: Who can the care-giver turn to for emotional support? The care-receiver?

A: People should find their support and their warm and empathetic relationships predominantly among their peers. It should not fall to one generation to meet the needs of another for affection, warmth, and support on an indefinite basis. If you have an elderly adult in the home, bring in people who are members of his peer group to become part of his support system. Move him out to them — take him to events and places where he may be with people who become his support system. This should be agreed to by you and your relative on a contractual basis. The care-giver may say, "I will be glad to have you living with me and as long as you are here these are the things I will do for you (cook, or arrange for mobile meals, etc.), but you must do your part, which will include arranging to go out twice a week to a social gathering."

Q: Can the care-giver prepare for crises?

A: We should anticipate that there will be crises and structure our relationships in such a way that those crises can be dealt with. We shouldn't anticipate that things will go badly. Generally, crises are little. A big crisis is something you cannot handle alone. If you wait long enough most crises will resolve themselves and sometimes working too hard at crisis resolution makes the crisis worse. You can build molehills into mountains. You have to identify the difference between a crisis of a small nature that will resolve and work itself out in time, and a crisis that is merely a symptom of a larger problem that has been unresolved for a long time and that needs to be worked on.

m. BOWING OUT

Most beginning care-givers have absolutely no idea of all the tasks involved in being the primary care-giver. Usually when they see the whole picture (it takes about two to three weeks) they almost give up the job but are persuaded to continue by their own desire to do "the right thing," plus the feeling of being wanted, needed, and appreciated by the care-receiver, other relatives, and the professionals. The care-receiver says, "I know I'm a lot of work — but I need you." Relatives tell you how wonderful you are, which makes you feel good and, of course, needed and useful. Nurses and community workers are delighted that you do everything they ask you and nod appreciatively when you tell them something new that helps the care-receiver feel better or respond better to treatment.

All of this is encouragement to continue taking on more and more; canceling more of your own regular activities; rushing more and sleeping less; doing what the care-receiver's doctor says and what the therapist or nurse says; until, gradually, you are spending all your time trying to give the care-receiver a good quality of life and the best nursing and social environment you know how to provide. But now you feel empty and disappointed.

Do not permit yourself to feel guilty for not having the stamina or heart to continue with the responsibility. You can regret not being able to continue without feeling guilty about it. Guilt and regret are not the same thing. Guilt is feeling that you did something you shouldn't have or didn't do something you should have. Regret is distress caused by the unpleasant realities of a situation.

Be honest with yourself and others — admit that you didn't expect things to be like this for so long, that you can't continue with the situation as it is. Then choose a method of ending or reducing your care-giving responsibilities so you can regain your stamina and social life, knowing that you gave proper notice and made arrangements for others to give appropriate and reliable help to the care-receiver.

The care-receiver's needs must be met by the community (society) in some way. (Food, shelter, clothing, and people are four of our basic needs.) The family care-giver usually feels that he or she provides an extra by helping. But the care-receiver's wants cannot enslave another and must be within the care-receiver's own financial means.

There are many ways to stop being the principal or main care-giver:

- You could die.
- You could get sick.
- You could have an accident.
- You could go away.
- You could walk out.
- Your care-receiver could fire you (even though you don't get paid).
- Your care-receiver could die.
- Your care-receiver could decide to have another relative arrange things for him or her.

Although these may seem a bit farfetched, they do happen; but there are better and more responsible ways to stop being the care-giver.

You could announce that you have decided not to do certain activities with or for the care-receiver, and that you will arrange for Mrs. Smith down the street, for example, to do them beginning next Thursday unless the care-receiver or other family members arrange something else that is agreeable to the care-receiver. If the care-receiver doesn't like your plan, explain that he or she is welcome to make other arrangements but that this arrangement is firm unless the care-receiver or other family members make another.

You could also tell the care-receiver's doctor that you will continue for the next two weeks only, but after that either the care-receiver or the doctor will have to make other arrangements.

You could place the care-receiver in a nursing home until arrangements are made for more permanent accommodation.

You could tell the community nurse or social worker that on the first Wednesday of next month you will be returning to your own home, and that as you have been unable to reassure the care-receiver that the person you wanted to ask to come in three days a week would be helpful, you are turning the help-in-house problem over to the nurse or social worker.

You could refuse to accept the responsibility of your relative's or spouse's care when the hospital tells you he or she is being discharged (for whatever reason). The hospital administration in cooperation with the community services should arrange for appropriate medical and accommodation care for the patient.

When you make arrangements for another care-giver to take over the responsibility of caring for your relative, be sure to set a date for the transfer. If for some reason the transfer date passes and you are unable to hand over the responsibility to a willing care-giver, notify the care-receiver's doctor, other relatives and/or the social worker of the situation. Tell them that if someone does not relieve you within 48 hours, you will hire a nurse at the care-receiver's expense or move your relative to a care facility, also at the care-receiver's expense. If after 48 hours there is still no willing care-giver, family or professional, then do what you said you would, notifying the care-receiver's doctor, one or two relatives, and the social worker you have been in communication with of the action you have taken.

There are rarely penalties for someone who must change plans for one reason or another, as long as adequate notice is given. If your priorities have changed and you feel that plans must be altered, you will suffer little financially. Remember, business people and creative people do it all the time. And criticism of your actions is not valid when and where your mental and physical health is concerned. You should not be pressured or encouraged to continue an activity that is causing you extreme stress. If your health is at risk of deteriorating, you must make changes in your life and daily routine to make sure that you stay healthy.

5

PROVIDING BETTER CARE

Most of us don't know enough about how our bodies work. The sections that follow highlight a few of the parts of the body, how they work, and what to do to keep them working.

Abusing the body is usually not done deliberately, but out of ignorance of the mechanics of the human being. Most popular publications on the newsstands carry at least one article on appearance, nutrition, or food. But how we see, hear, walk, and use or abuse medicines are not as commonly featured. They are important.

After reading the following information on the problems of some older people, you'll be better prepared to help your partner or relative live as comfortable a life as possible.

A few doctors and nurses tend to consider signs, symptoms, and the discomfort of their patient only in the context of the primary diagnosis. For example, an irritated nose may not be considered important enough for treatment because the patient has severe heart problems. Tiredness and sluggishness may be considered not worth investigating if the patient has had a stroke.

An excuse can always be made that the person is old or has high blood pressure or arthritis or cancer or some other condition or disease. But if the patient didn't, the symptoms would be investigated and an attempt would be made to make him or her more comfortable.

Unless medical personnel try to alleviate day-to-day discomforts, dissatisfaction arises on the part of the care-giver and discomfort continues for the patient, which diminishes the quality of life.

The present is very important when one has a chronic disorder or a serious illness. If your relative is not enjoying today because of some physical discomfort, that must be dealt with. If the problem cannot be removed, the chronically ill patient must be taught pain management techniques so that discomfort can be endured. And the terminally ill person must be assisted in gaining comfort using techniques developed by medical teams working in hospice programs providing care for the dying.

a. EYES

Sight impairment and other eye problems are usually observed and treated quickly by doctors, but it is wise to have regular eye examinations to make sure that vision is being assisted by the most appropriate lenses (either contacts or glasses).

Eye examinations should be done more frequently when a person has a chronic disorder. Too often there is a tendency for a few well-meaning professionals and family care-givers to automatically assume that problems such as stumbling, bumping into things, and misinterpreting directions on prescription labels are related to the care-receiver's disorder. Ordinarily, poor sight would be one of the first explanations considered if the person experiencing these problems was reasonably healthy. But because a person has a chronic illness or progressive disorder, many care-providers think that eye problems, or other symptoms that could indicate eye problems (such as being vague, failing to take medicine at the right time, not being able to dial the phone correctly) are probably part of the disease and must simply be accepted.

This may not be the case. Eye changes are common in people over 40. It is wise, therefore, to have an eye checkup every year.

For people who have difficulty reading, it is helpful to choose printed material which has print 9 point or larger. (Point size is how printers measure type size. The print in this book is 12 point. Print that is 9 point is slightly smaller.) Material should also be black print on white paper, rounded letters, primarily lower-case type (lower-case is easier to read than upper-case), a lot of white around the letter and the word, and space between paragraphs and short lines as in newspaper style.

b. FEET

Some concerns to care-receivers are corns, calluses, warts, ingrown toenails, thick skin, fungus disorders, infections, itchy skin, dryness, numbness, rash between toes, sores, sensitive feet, hot feet, tingling, tenderness, and bunions.

Most of these conditions can be treated and, in some cases, prevented. Almost all can be alleviated to make wearing shoes more comfortable and walking easier.

To correct a foot problem, begin by having a medical examination. If treatment is suggested, follow through. Also, make sure that shoes are suitable and fit well. Shoes should be kept in good repair; pay special attention to heels wearing down. Socks and stockings should fit well — not too tight or too loose. Allow time for proper foot care on a regular basis (e.g., dry well between toes). And finally, gather information on the care of the feet and skin.

c. TEETH AND DENTURES*

Rare is the older person who still has every original tooth in place. Even more rare is the older person who has never had a filling or a tooth extracted.

We look at our teeth every day in the mirror, from the crowns to the gums. But we can't see what's inside or see the roots imbedded in the gums.

The nerve canal is the sensitive part of every tooth. When the dentist does a root canal, that's where he or she is working.

Next time you look at your teeth, give an extra look at your gums. They are likely to be healthy if they are tight around your teeth and are a light-pink, stippled color. Between your teeth, the gums should come to a point where the teeth touch.

Around each tooth and attached to the jaw-bone, is the periodontal membrane. It is the holder-in-place; it's like living elastic, truly wonderful!

1. Toothaches

Many young people have not had the experience of a toothache. On the other hand, it's an exceptional old-timer who hasn't had a dandy!

Toothaches are simple affairs! They happen when infection or an irritant gets to the nerve through a cavity. Toothaches also happen when pus forms at the root and makes an abscess.

Here are some of the organisms and substances that affect our teeth negatively:

- Bacteria generate acid that dissolves the enamel and root cementum. Bacteria can then infect and destroy the tooth.

---

* This information originally appeared in the April 1980 "Pioneer News," a Bank of British Columbia newsletter for senior citizens. It is reprinted here with the kind permission of journalist Chuck Bayley and the Bank of British Columbia.

- Infection generates pus that creates pressure at the root of the tooth, as an abscess.
- Gum disease works on the periodontal membrane, thus weakening its hold on the teeth.
- Foreign materials cause stain! It's easy to see dark brown tobacco stain; yellow plaque (plak) stain; and blue mineral dust stain.
- Constant grinding (even when we are asleep) wears down the biting surfaces.
- Harsh cleaning substances and heavy scrubbing harm the teeth.

Teeth are hard and tough; however, they cannot withstand everything that comes at them or sticks to them. They need your own personal attention. That means cleaning, flossing, and rinsing.

2. Plaque

Dentists and dental hygienists make a lot of fuss about plaque. That's because it's a serious problem; it harbors tooth-destroying elements.

Soft plaque is a sticky, bacteria-ridden film that gathers on teeth at the inside and outside gum lines, and also between the teeth. If we allow it to stay and stick, the plaque gets thicker, infects the gums, and breaks down the enamel.

Hard plaque, sometimes called calculus or tartar, is a mineral deposit that adheres to teeth. It irritates the gums and particularly the periodontal (holding) membrane.

There's only one way to beat plaque, and that's by regular and correct cleaning. If you do not keep your teeth free of plaque, ultimately you will have to get your dentist or hygienist to remove it.

3. Mouth troubles

We don't often think of what can go wrong inside our mouths. Here are some examples of what can:

- Gum recession tends to come with aging, especially if teeth have been neglected. In this, the gums no longer cover the roots.
- Bone recession also comes with aging, and the bone, which supports the teeth, is lost. This occurs more often under dentures.

- Dry-mouth, or xerostomia, happens when insufficient saliva is flowing. It tends to come with age and with body upset. Denture wearers experience it more often than others do. Generally, the healthier your body, the better the saliva flow.
- Periodontal disease is the destruction of the periodontal membrane by infection. It's commonly called pyorrhea.
- Lip cracks are caused by overclosing, which comes when the tooth surfaces wear down and form nutrition deficiencies and disease.
- Sense of taste declines with age, starting at about age 50. Smokers and denture wearers are more affected than others.
- Burning tongue is caused by irritants, allergies, and diet deficiencies. Denture wearers may have this problem when their bite is overclosed.
- Jaw-joint stiffening is often an arthritic condition. Movement is limited and this causes discomfort. Chewing helps to keep your jaws working!
- Gingivitis is an infection. The gums redden, swell and bleed easily. Regular cleaning and a nutritious diet are the best ways to avoid gingivitis.
- Lumps, spots, and sores can occur in your mouth for many reasons. If you notice any, see your dentist.

Have your mouth checked periodically to make certain there's no trouble inside. That's professional advice.

4. Give teeth care

The best way to keep out of the dentist's chair is to take care of your teeth. The rules are clean and simple: use fluorides; brush and rinse well at least once a day; eat a low-sugar, nutritious diet; and see your dentist at regular intervals.

Plaque is the number one enemy of your teeth, so fight it. Use a small, soft toothbrush with nylon bristles; use fluoride toothpaste, dental floss, and disclosing tablets.

Use the "wiggle" motion in brushing. Have the bristles at a 45 degree angle and direct them toward the gumline. Apply enough pressure to allow the bristles to go just under the gums. "Wiggle" the brush, at least to the count of ten. Do two or three teeth at a time. That loosens the plaque and you can sweep it away with your brush.

5. Dentures take care

Surprise! Dentures require attention; they affect health and comfort. Care means cleaning every day; it means professional cleaning, periodically; it means having repairs and relines done professionally when they are needed.

- Remove your dentures overnight and put them to soak in water. If you do not like to have them out overnight, at least remove them for a few hours during the day and soak them in water. Your gums deserve a rest!
- Rinse your dentures under warm water after every meal and rinse your mouth.
- Brush your dentures once a day, well, using a soft brush with toothpaste or soap and water.
- Brush your tongue and gums, and rinse your mouth before replacing your dentures.

It's good advice to see your dentist regularly for a check of your mouth and dentures.

Don't expect your dentures to fit perfectly forever; your gums and supporting structure will shrink.

Don't try yourself to make them fit using a do-it-yourself kit. The risk is too great and you can easily cause open sores. See your dentist or denturist.

If you break your dentures, take them to your dentist or denturist to be repaired. You can easily damage them and irritate your mouth.

If your dentures are fitting well and everything inside is healthy, you should be able to eat and speak comfortably. There's no better test!

6. Care for partials

Some partials stay in place, others come out. Both types require care, as do the abutment teeth to which they are attached and the gums underneath. If the anchor teeth go, that's the end of the partial plate.

Cleaning a removal partial is the same as a full denture: brushing, soaking, rinsing. The partial must be handled gently so as not to bend or fracture the clamps or bars.

The surrounding natural teeth require thorough cleaning in the usual way: brushing and flossing.

Even with a partial denture, your gums need a rest. Leave it out for two or three hours at a time, in water or in the solution.

Bridges have their own problems because they stay in place. It's more difficult to clean the anchor teeth and gums; your dentist should show you how. You can use floss, knitting yarn, interprosimal tips, and a special brush. Your dentist might recommend a water irrigation device.

Clean the anchor teeth gently; avoid any abrasive pressure on the tooth surface below the metal crowns.

7. Food for teeth

From infancy, even from the prenatal stage, nutrition affects our teeth, gums, bone structure, and general health of our mouths, throughout life. We must continually give attention to what we eat and drink.

The following are to be noted:

- Burning tongue and cracks at the corner of the mouth might be related to lack of vitamin B in your diet.
- Bleeding gums might be due to insufficient vitamin C.
- Lessening of bone density and the development of osteoporosis might be signs of not enough calcium, vitamin D, and fluoride.

These discomforts can be avoided, to a large extent, by adhering to a nutritious diet. We tend to overlook this requirement as we get older.

The [Canada] Food Guide gives the four essential groups of food that provide us with the correct balance of foods on a daily basis. You can obtain much information on food requirements from your local community public health office. However, consult your dentist if your teeth or mouth are giving you trouble.

These are the four food groups in the Food Guide:

- milk and milk products (2 servings per day)
- meat and alternatives (2 servings per day)
- bread and cereals (3 to 5 servings per day)
- fruit and vegetables (4 to 5 servings per day)

8. Eating and dentures

First-time denture wearers are likely to have some difficulty in biting, chewing, and swallowing in a coordinated action. For these persons, biting can be difficult; chewing, not quite as difficult; swallowing, the easiest.

Again from the experience of many, we can say it's best to keep away from sandwiches and raw vegetables, at first. When you can tackle these without difficulty, you have triumphed.

If you continue to experience discomfort, go back to where you obtained your dentures and have the fitting checked. Some persons change their diet to try and cure the problem; that's a mistake. Seniors need to be able to eat good protein, vegetables, fruits: less fats, starches, and sugars.

d. EARS AND HEARING AIDS*

1. How the system works

The outer ear funnels in the sound waves. These strike the ear drum which is a tight membrane stretched across the inner end of the ear canal.

This striking causes the three connected bones in the inner ear to move — to carry the vibrations. The bone attached to the ear drum is the malleus (hammer). The middle bone is the incus (anvil). The innermost bone is the stapes (stirrup); it fits into the opening to the inner ear.

The inner ear is filled with fluid. The snail-like (cochlea) portion of the inner ear contains many fine hairs that are connected to special cells.

The vibrations, which come by means of the three connected bones, cause motion within the fluid. This makes the hairs move, which causes the cells to send electrical impulses along the auditory nerve to the brain.

In the brain, the electrical impulses produce sensations that we know as sounds. In some mysterious way, these sounds become meaningful to us.

---

*This information is reprinted from the "Pioneer News," August/September 1979, with the kind permission of Chuck Bayley and the Bank of British Columbia.

2. Causes of hearing loss

In the outer ear, wax might be blocking the passage; if so, your physician can remove it. Other blockages might require surgery.

In the middle ear, the lining might become infected or the ear drum damaged by a sudden loud noise or by an extreme change in air pressure. The three middle ear bones might become immobilized or disconnected and lose their ability to transmit vibrations.

In the inner ear, damage to the delicate nerve system could be permanent because, to date, there is no way to repair sensori-nerve loss.

Here are the common causes of nerve loss, some of which can be prevented:

- Hereditary factors
- Diseases, such as German measles, contracted by the mother during the early months of pregnancy
- Perinatal problems such as prematurity.
- Certain drugs such as some antibiotics, quinine, and diuretics.
- Meniere's Disease, which produces extra fluid in the inner ear. This causes dizziness, head noises, and hearing loss. In many cases, it can be treated successfully
- Circulation problems, head injuries, and tumors.
- Exposure to intense sounds. This loss might happen so gradually that it might not be noticed for years
- Aging, which reduces the ability to hear high-pitched sounds and to understand what is being said

Sometimes a person is unaware that a hearing loss is taking place, but other members of the family notice. The person should be encouraged, not forced, to see the doctor.

3. Signs of difficulty

These are several warning signals:

- Familiar sounds might not seem as loud as usual
- Conversation, especially in a group, might be difficult to make out
- High-pitched sounds, such as a clock ticking or the phone ringing, might be missed

- There might be a hissing or ringing sound that seems to come from the ear or head

These difficulties tend to make you feel uneasy, even irritable, and wonder what is happening. The rule is, "Consult your physician without delay." If the problem requires further medical investigation, your physician will refer you to an ear specialist.

If your hearing loss cannot be corrected by medical means, then you should consider buying a hearing aid.

You must understand that a "hearing aid" is an "aid to hearing." It cannot restore or produce natural hearing.

You must also accept the fact that you have to learn how to handle and take care of your hearing aid. That won't be a new experience; we all have learned to operate various types of electronic devices.

Hearing aids have four basic components. Some have extra features. Some are more suited to particular hearing problems.

These are the four basic components:

- A tiny microphone that picks up the sound and changes it into impulses.
- An amplifier that increases the strength of the impulses, with a battery providing the power.
- A receiver that changes the stepped-up impulses back into sound.
- An earmold that directs the sound into the ear canal and then on through the hearing system. The earmold should be custom-made and fit your ear properly. If it doesn't, you will get feedback whistle or squeal.

There are four types of hearing aids:

- In-the-ear hearing aids fit into the ear, almost flush.
- Behind-the-ear hearing aids are worn behind the ear. A short plastic tube connects the case and the earmold.
- On-the-body hearing aids are attached to the clothing or carried in a pocket. This type is usually more powerful. The case and earmold are connected by a cord.
- Eyeglass hearing aids have the amplifier built into the temple of the frame. A short plastic tube connects the case and earmold.

4. Buying a hearing aid

You have been checked by your physician and by an ear specialist or a qualified audiologist. You are advised that hearing aid seems advisable. Then, what do you do?

This advice is offered:

- Never buy a hearing aid through mail-order, and stay clear of out-of-state or out-of-province special offers.
- Do not go directly to a hearing aid dealer or to a professional audiologist; see your doctor first.
- No two people have identical hearing. A hearing aid that suits a friend might not suit you. Take professional advice.
- Remember you are free to shop around until you are satisfied as to service, quality, guarantee, and price.
- Before you say, "Yes, I'll take it," and before you sign an agreement to buy, obtain in writing the itemized cost, free service provided, guarantee, trial period, and refund policy.
- Most dealers allow for a trial period. However, expect a charge to cover the cost of the work done, if you return the hearing aid within the trial period.

5. The way to start

It takes time and a bit of learning to become accustomed to a hearing aid. Several million persons have succeeded, so your chances should be good.

Conscientious dealers and clinics carefully show how to use and how to care for the hearing aid. You should expect this service.

(a) Tell your friends and family how your hearing aid works. Tell them they can help — by getting your attention before they start to talk; by facing you when they speak; by talking normally without shouting, but speaking more slowly and clearly.

(b) Start using your hearing aid around the house for short periods to get used to the new sound. Start talking with one person at home; stand or sit fairly close, facing each other.

(c) Gradually expand the situations so you encounter more sounds. It helps to note the action taking place. Be ready to adjust the volume so you can hear comfortably.

(d) Consider learning to lip-read. It's a useful skill for everyone.

As for the telephone, hold the hearing end up to the microphone of your hearing aid and it will pick up the voice.

6. Tips on care

- Handle your hearing aid gently. Don't knock or drop it.
- Keep the earmold dry and clean.
- Detach the earmold regularly and wash it. Use a mild soap and water or a recommended cleaner.
- Never clean with alcohol or tetrachloride.
- If the opening in the earmold becomes clogged with wax, remove it gently using a toothpick.
- Take care not to puncture the earmold or the tubing.
- Dry the earmold well before reattaching it to the tubing. Watch for tiny bubbles of water in the tube. Shake or blow them out.
- Keep your hearing aid away from heat. That means out of the sun and away from the stove and heater. The glove compartment of your car is not a good place, either.
- Remove your hearing aid before applying hair spray. It can damage the microphone.
- Read about the care of batteries in the booklet that comes with your hearing aid. Remember, batteries provide the power to make your hearing aid work. Learn how to put the battery in and take it out. Find out how to keep the contact points bright and clean. Turn off your hearing aid when you are not using it. Remove the battery at night. Most important and not to be forgotten, keep a fresh spare battery on hand. Throw away old batteries.

Have your hearing aid and earmold serviced regularly.

- Do not try to repair your hearing aid yourself because it is delicate and intricate.
- For servicing and repairing, take it where you bought it.

7. Questions and good answers

Q: How can I stop feeling embarrassed when wearing my hearing aid?

A: Thousands of people wear hearing aids, so they don't carry a stigma. Once you discover the advantages of your aid, you will forget it is in place, except when you stop to appreciate its benefits.

Share information about your hearing aid with your family and friends; some day they might need one.

Q: Why do background noises come in louder?

A: The hearing aid picks up and amplifies all sounds. You must concentrate on what you want to hear. If this doesn't help, go back to where you bought your aid and explain your problem. Some minor adjustment might be needed.

Q: How do I reduce clothing noises?

A: This happens only with on-the-body type hearing aids. Clothing in contact with the aid should be soft. You can get a special carrier garment.

Q: What if the earmold hurts?

A: Do not accept or wear an earmold that hurts. Go back to where you bought your hearing aid; the earmold might have to be remade.

Q: What if my behind-the-ear feels bulky?

A: It should fit comfortably because it is light and contoured. Give yourself time to get used to it. Then, if it doesn't feel right, go back to where you bought it and have the fitting checked.

Q: Why do people tend to shout when they notice the hearing aid?

A: They think they are helping you and do not know a hearing aid amplifies sounds. Just tell them to speak in a normal voice.

Q: Why are there differences in the cost of hearing aids?

A: Hearing aids are no different from any other product. The cost depends on the type, design, style, quality, and service. The cost includes the hearing aid itself, testing, fitting, counselling, after-purchase service, guarantee, and overhead. As a buyer, it is up to you to get the best value for your money and to be satisfied.

Q: What do you do about radio and TV?

A: Sit eight to ten feet away from the set. If your hearing aid has a tone control, adjust it until you get the most pleasant sound. Listen to the rhythm and pace of the sound. That helps you to follow the action and meaning with greater ease.

You can buy an ear plug that will plug into your radio and TV. Head sets with a volume control are also available.

8. Quick checks

If a hearing aid is not working —

(a) Try a fresh battery. Make certain it is placed properly in the battery compartment.

(b) Check the tubing. A sharp bend or kink blocks the sound.

(c) Check the earmold. It might be blocked with wax.

(d) Try your spare cord if yours is an on-the-body aid. The other might have a break.

(e) If you have a telephone pick-up on your aid, check the switch. It could be in the T-position.

If sound comes on and off, or is scratchy —

(a) Turn your switch on and off several times. There might be a bit of dust or lint.

(b) If an on-the-body aid, push the cord plugs in and out several times; they might not be making a good connection. Or try your spare cord.

If whistling —

(a) Remove your hearing aid from your ear. If the whistling increases, put your finger over the opening of the earmold. If the whistling then stops, you did not have the earmold in your ear properly, or it is a poor fit.

(b) If whistling keeps on when you have your finger over the earmold opening, take the hearing aid back to where you bought it for a check.

Hearing is precious; take good care of it. When it is not working well, get professional advice, the sooner the better.

e. MEDICATION

Medicines, commonly called drugs by doctors, nurses, and pharmacists (not to be confused with illegal drugs), can be either prescription drugs, signed for by your doctor, or over-the-counter drugs (non-prescription medicine), which merely means you buy them the way you buy any other item for personal use. But sometimes medications, either prescriptions or over-the-counter, can become ineffective or make you ill when taken with other drugs and foods.

The Ten Commandments of drug use contain sound advice:*

THOU SHALT: Consult your doctor about the name and purpose of your medication

THOU SHALT: Inform your doctor about all medication, pills, potions or lotions you may be taking, old or new.

THOU SHALT: Seek a professional service from only one pharmacy and choose one that keeps a patient record card of all your medications and over-the-counter drugs.

THOU SHALT: Take your medication as directed: the right dose, at the right time, in the right way and for the prescribed length of time. Always keep your medication in its original labelled container, in a cool, dry place.

THOU SHALT: Use exercise, good food, and a positive attitude to develop a healthy lifestyle.

THOU SHALT NOT: Take pills that you only recognize by color or shape.

THOU SHALT NOT: Hoard, borrow, lend, or substitute medication of any kind.

THOU SHALT NOT: Shop around for drugs like one does for groceries.

THOU SHALT NOT: Double dose missed doses; stop treatment in mid-stream or take other substitutes without informing your doctor or pharmacy; nor should you mix pills or put them in unlabelled containers.

THOU SHALT NOT: Substitute a pill for all of life's ills.

f. HEALTH INSURANCE

Like a will or funeral and burial arrangements, you don't have to have health insurance. Neither does your care-receiver. Although it is not required by law, having health insurance is both practical and prudent.

If your employer offers an extended (additional) health benefit plan covering such medical expenses as nurses, ambulance, physiotherapy, etc., do consider accepting the offer. Employers usually pay about half or more of the premium. Some plans are effective even if you are unable to work again or are retired.

---

*These Ten Commandments of drug use were originally formulated by the Medications Awareness Group, Vancouver, British Columbia.

Another insurance to consider is income replacement insurance. If you hold such a policy and become ill and unable to work for a while, you will receive a specific amount of income until you are able to resume work.

g. CREATE A MINI-BIOGRAPHY

Ensuring that your relative gets the best care possible includes helping the care professionals to become knowledgeable about the care-receiver. To do this, prepare a list of the care-receiver's interests and a sort of mini-biography (see Worksheet #11). Most of the agencies you will be dealing with already have, or will insist on knowing, the main medical information and vital statistics, but they rarely ask about the things that make life important to all of us — our feelings, opinions, activities, family, and friends. You can use this as a guide or write a biography yourself. Put in only those things that the care-receiver feels are important. He or she will have been talking about or doing some of them during the past year. After you've jotted down a few things about your relative you can ask other family members to add things they feel the care-receiver thinks are important. If the care-receiver is rational and has the energy, he or she may want to fill in the blanks personally or help suggest additions to the biography.

A person's life is a good deal more than his or her vital statistics and medical history. Doctors, nurses, and other staff members at care facilities should also know some of the care-receiver's likes, dislikes, preferences, and past and present interests. Mention and talk about places your relative has travelled; involvement in clubs, sports, or hobbies; any awards received; participation in or survivor or witness of events such as war, earthquake, tornado, or train wreck; first person to do or see something; his or her former profession; and so on.

The more the staff and professionals know about the patient and your concerns, the harder it will be for them to remain indifferent and superficial. You and your care-receiver must volunteer this information, making sure not to disclose private information that your relative does not want revealed. Your efforts will encourage professionals and volunteers to take the personal risk of becoming more involved, more understanding, and more straightforward.

A review of life interests shows care-receivers as unique individuals. Patients cannot be merely room numbers or cases when looked at in this way. Paint a composite picture of your spouse or relative so that others do not see him or her only as "the person in Room 4 with the stroke whose relative visits each day." You want them to think, for example, "That is Mr. Jones, 73 years old, who speaks two languages, who not long ago completed a consulting job with an overseas firm. He became widowed five months ago. His wife was his sole companion and best friend."

WORKSHEET #11
OUTLINE FOR MINI-BIOGRAPHY

MINI-BIOGRAPHY
of _____

Prepared by _____
Date _____

1. Talks about (e.g., people, places, events)
2. Favorite colors   sounds
   fragrances   clothes
   foods   furniture
3. Interests
4. Hobbies and leisure activities
5. Jobs — past, recently and present
6. Towns and countries worked in
7. Languages familiar with or spoken fluently
8. Accomplishments, school, skills, courses taken or being taken now
9. Experiences (e.g., when young, on the farm, during the war, when travelling, at first job, etc.)
10. Vital statistics
    Born: when, where
    Married: to, when
    Children: names
11. Medical history: especially the times in hospital or off work due to illness, injuries on the job or off, etc.

6
PROBLEM AREAS

Most of the concerns discussed in this chapter will be yours at some point in your care-giving experience. You will deal with each one as it comes up and will probably not have to consider it a problem again. I have included this material because care-givers don't usually have the luxury of free time to consider solutions once a problem is apparent.

There are many problems that could occur in your job as care-giver. You could be distrusted, be left out of the will, or spend many nights in hospital waiting rooms waiting to hear the latest report of your care-receiver's condition. You may even have to be almost torn away from caring for your relative and allow someone else to take over because — believe it or not — you may not recognize that you cannot, anymore, give the kind of care your relative needs. You may have exhausted yourself to the point where you need relief from the 24-hour responsibility.

Some awful things can happen. If you know about them, you'll be better prepared to cope.

a. TRUST

Obstacles to trust are generally in the heart, habits, and experiences of the care-receiver. The care-receiver may never trust you — not because of anything you have done, but because at some time in the past someone your relative trusted handled a situation unsatisfactorily and the memory is still very strong. The fact that it was another person, another time, another place, and probably a different set of circumstances doesn't seem to take away the care-receiver's feelings of distrust, hesitancy, and fear.

Whether the care-receiver trusts you or not, you can still be the care-giver. The care-receiver may want you to be the care-giver even under these circumstances. This is a particularly difficult situation — you are wanted, but not for some things.

Whenever possible, get another person who is trusted to do the tasks the care-receiver doesn't want you to do. Some of the things your relative may not trust you to do include dressings, treatments, irrigations, dialysis, helping him or her walk, pushing the wheelchair, banking, or taking care of legal matters.

Although you may feel hurt that your relative does not trust you in certain areas, you should recognize that this is a common problem and does not necessarily reflect poorly on your abilities.

b. SLIGHT GRADUAL CHANGES

Changes in a care-receiver's condition are sometimes difficult to detect if the care-giver sees the spouse or relative on a daily basis. If a change is gradual, because you see the person constantly you may not be aware of a change in condition until the situation becomes a crisis.

You should not panic or feel guilty, thinking that you may have been negligent or at fault. Naturally, you do your best to notice changes in your relative, but sometimes these happen almost imperceptibly and are more easily recognized by others who see the care-receiver only occasionally.

c. TIME

Some concerns and considerations about time are —

- How long can you expect the family, friends, and yourself to help?
- How long are friends willing to wait for you to become available to them like you used to be?
- How long will the care-receiver's friends wait around for their friend to resume being his or her old self and to do things with them again?
- How long will the care-receiver's friends continue to visit?
- How long is long?

Some care-givers are bitter, angry, and disappointed that they are too busy to take part in discussions, learn new methods, make more thorough arrangements, develop contingency plans, go more places, and do more things. They feel they have no time of their own and no one to relieve them. They don't even have time to find out if there is anyone who could take over for a while. They won't take the time to teach someone to help ("easier to do it myself") and think it is too much trouble to make arrangements for a temporary relief companion just to go to a few hours' lecture ("I'd rather not go out").

Care-givers also frequently feel very disorganized, even though they are probably more organized than ever before. Friends say, "But your house is always so clean and tidy!" Trying to be prepared for an emergency is always on the care-giver's mind. The housekeeping, cleaning, tidying, and dishes seem to be never-ending. The care-giver keeps train and bus schedules handy, knows the phone number for a taxi by heart, knows to the hour when medicine refills are to be ordered, and has extra basic foods stocked, just in case. One care-giver knows where all the telephone booths are between his house and his parents even though he has a car phone.

Time is the precious commodity care-givers always want more of to accomplish all they wish to do.

Knowing where you spend your time and how much of your time is spent on priority activities is the first step to using your time more efficiently. Review the section on time management in chapter 4 and fill out the activity assessment sheets every few weeks. Make your life more satisfying by finding time for yourself so you will not have nagging regrets that you chose to be a care-giver. Filling some of your wants and all of your needs will ensure that you have the emotional and physical resources to share, give, and care for another.

Establish realistic priorities for yourself and for your involvement with the care-receiver. Identify and eliminate your time-wasting activities (only you can say what you consider time-wasters), and control and prevent unwanted interruptions. For example, establish a policy for visitors' calls — in person and by telephone — and for calls by salespeople and repair technicians.

If you control your life and activities instead of allowing yourself to be controlled by others, you will have time to do what you want.

d. JOB HINDRANCES

These are the main problems that prevent care-givers from doing as thorough and effective a job as they would like:

(a) Not being recognized as the care-receiver's coordinator and the reporter to the rest of the family (with the care-receiver's approval, of course)

(b) Frequently lacking essential information

(c) Not being extended normal business and professional courtesy (i.e., appointments, phone calls, letters, printed directions and explanations, regular meetings, consideration of your time and schedule, assistance with priorities and decision-making when hesitant or requesting assistance, etc.)

(d) Rarely having time to learn to be a better care-giver and coordinator — taking courses, reading, viewing instructive films, participating in workshops suitable for expressing concerns and sharing ideas — and not being given sufficient useful printed material to reflect upon and then try out suggested remedies during the infrequent periods between essential tasks and crises.

(e) Not feeling able to truly communicate with professionals, bureaucrats, other family members, and the care-receiver.

(f) Doing little or no long-term planning — even two weeks ahead.

(g) Not having contingency plans for minor happenings in the normal course of events. Perhaps the neighbor forgets she has promised to drive the care-receiver to the doctor. Or after a 45-minute wait the receptionist says the doctor has been detained at the hospital and won't be able to keep the appointment. Such minor problems can become crises if the care-giver is unable to handle unexpected changes in plans.

(h) Not having enough time to themselves.

(i) Feeling unhappy or uncertain about their own role and dealing with the negative or unhelpful attitudes of some relatives, friends, and professional service providers.

e. RECOGNITION

Care-givers want recognition for what they do. Those who effectively juggle their own lives, their families' activities, and the extra arrangements for the infirm or ill relative do not feel they need constant verbal praise. However, there is a tendency for some care-givers to compete with one another when talking about how much harder it is to cope with their relative than it is with other care-givers' relatives. What these care-givers really want is to be told they are doing a good job without having to beg.

Care-givers do like to share ideas of management. But poor management, poor time use, failing to look after oneself mentally and physically, and failing to have a life of one's own should not be rewarded with sympathy.

When you visit or telephone someone, do not talk only about the care-receiver. Encourage conversation about what's new, the movie on TV last night, etc. By taking the focus off the care-receiver you can feel that you are a whole person, not just the relative of whomever you are caring for.

It is also important that you have someone to confide in, someone who is either not connected with the care-receiver or who, although involved, can look at the situation objectively. Verbalizing your feelings helps you to put them in perspective; talking about problems, frustrations, hopes, and needs help you to see the situation more clearly.

Care-givers need a sounding board, not someone who will tell them what to do. Care-givers need friends who care about them as individuals.

f. WAITING

Waiting is difficult, and as a care-giver it may seem that you are waiting for just about everything: waiting for the next crisis, waiting for phone calls, waiting for information, waiting to talk to the doctor, waiting for an appointment, waiting for the end, waiting for your own life to resume, waiting for the next treatment, waiting for the treatment to be finished, waiting for the results, waiting for a more normal time, and so on.

Waiting is not always procrastination. Neither is hesitation necessarily procrastination. It may be that you do not have all the information you need to proceed further. But if you defer a decision or course of action, you should have a reason for doing so.

You should also have a reason for waiting and an idea of how long you are willing to wait. If you are bothered by the waiting, set a time limit to it: "I will worry about that for five minutes and no more," or, "I will stay here for ten minutes longer and if I don't get my appointment I will leave," or, "I will make a decision on Wednesday based on the information I have at that time. A decision must be made, as I can't go through life constantly waiting for more information. I can always change my decision later if circumstances change or new information comes to my attention."

g. THE SWEET CARE-RECEIVER

One of the least talked about frustrations of being a care-giver is caring for care-receivers who never complain and are constantly grateful and appreciative. The care-giver says, "How can I complain about sweetness?"

These care-receivers say things like, "Hope I'm no trouble." If you say they are but you wouldn't be helping them if you didn't want to, they counter with, "I don't want to be a bother," or, "You do so much for me," or, "I won't get in your way...you do what you have to do...I'll watch," or, "I'll go into the other room so you can work — I don't want to be a nuisance."

Actually, these people are delightful and we love them, but as these conversations occur day in and day out the care-giver begins to think he or she is going crazy. And then a care-giver may feel guilty for resenting the "appreciative" compliments.

The helpless, "Poor me...I wish I were able to do more so you wouldn't have to do this for me" is a common form of expression you hear when you first become the care-giver. Perhaps for the first month or so you appreciate it, but from then on the care-receiver is usually merely mouthing words that he or she noticed you received gratefully and responded to by reaffirming your willingness to help. The care-receiver has been allowed to continue using these phrases until they have become a habit. The care-receiver is rewarded for saying them by being talked to and reassured that he or she is loved and "can't help" being old or having a chronic disorder or being handicapped and requiring assistance.

It is very difficult to halt this habit if it is long standing or if the person had the manipulative "you do so much for me" behavior before becoming disabled, chronically ill, or frail. There is no easy way of explaining that this type of conversation is irritating you to the point where you stiffen when your relative approaches because you are anticipating the "Sigh, sigh, ho, hum...making my lunch? Wonderful...I am so lucky to have you...you are so good to me. I wonder what other people do who don't have such wonderful daughters..."

Tell your relative how you feel about this type of verbal gratitude — once or twice. If he or she continues, it could be that he or she forgets or doesn't believe that it bothers you.

It is a difficult situation. There are some care-givers who are criticized from morning till night by their care-receivers and family and would love to hear a word of appreciation — at least once — and never get it.

h. REPETITIOUS CHATTER AND INTERRUPTIONS

Constant repetitious chatter is also a frustrating problem for the care-giver.

Again, there is no easy solution and sometimes there is no solution at all. You can avoid chatter occasionally by going out or arranging for your relative to go out. Also, with cooperation you can say, for example, "Not now, Mother. I am doing the books — we'll talk later."

If you are interrupted constantly, you may decide that it is a nervous habit. If so, you'll have to take more breaks away from the chatterer who insists on a reply from you. You could establish places in the house where the chatterer knows you do not appreciate being spoken to, or where you can't easily respond over the noise of, for example, the washing machine, dryer, or lawnmower.

But do try to hold the care-receiver's attention long enough, a few times, to make it clear that you are interested in him or her but that there are times when you would rather not talk or even listen.

i. THE UNREASONABLE CARE-RECEIVER

"I will come and look after you for a few days after you get out of the hospital, Mother," you say.

"Then how will I manage?" she asks.

"The doctor is arranging for the community nurse to come see you to help us decide what you will need."

"I don't want strangers around. We don't know them — they might steal something."

"We may have to take that chance, Mom, but don't forget that anyone who steals will lose his or her job for sure."

"I don't care — I won't have strangers about."

"They are only strangers, Mom, until you get to know them."

"Well, I won't have it."

This is a useless conversation, and if you continue it you are being as unreasonable as your mother is. The family, in the above example, cannot humor mother indefinitely just because she is timid and reluctant to have outside help and/or employees. You must let her know that although you are quite prepared to help, you are not going to be inconvenienced unreasonably.

You may dislike housework and be unwilling to do your mother's, while your sister might like housework but be unwilling to take your Mom to the hospital for treatments, which you don't mind doing at all. And if neither of you wants to move in with Mom or have her move in with you, you must consider alternatives, which might include some free community help, paid housekeeping and gardening, etc.

j. SELFISHNESS

Some people think that selfishness is thinking of yourself to the exclusion of others. Yes, but...

Some people think that unselfishness is putting your time and energies at the disposal of their demands and desires — doing what they want and not necessarily what is good for you or what you want to do. In other words, if you follow their wishes you are unselfish; if you don't, you are selfish. Actually, it is they who are selfish for wanting you to martyr yourself to their wants.

Some people think that inconveniences, suffering, and martyrdom are good for the soul, build moral fiber, and make you a good person.

That is rot. If some people do improve under all the stress, it is because they had the soul and fiber in the first place. Too often, unfortunately, people who are "compelled" to do things they find inconvenient or assume roles that cause them to suffer become bitter, critical, and dissatisfied with nearly everything. A bitter person is not a pleasant person to have out for the evening, yet angry, bitter people often wonder why they don't have many friends.

Do not allow yourself to become a martyr. Taking your own mental and physical health into account is not an act of selfishness.

k. LOSSES AND ANTICIPATORY GRIEF

We suffer when relatives and those we care about lose vitality, livelihood, health, or the ability to communicate easily. It is not unusual to grieve over something gone or something going but not yet gone. This sense of loss is a fact, it is stressful, and it is uncomfortable. It is normal to feel sad when losing something we are used to or someone we love.

You may miss the qualities, expressions, and presence of your relative and mourn the loss even when he or she is still in the same house with you. This sense of loss is similar to the loss suffered by the bereaved, and you will probably feel peculiar to miss these things when the care-receiver is still alive and may be alive for months or many years. It is as if it is improper to "feel" before a person dies and to grieve now for the things the care-receiver can no longer do or is pretending he or she can still do but performs badly: communicating; looking after him or herself; sharing decisions about banking, changes in accommodation, gifts for others; arguing about grandson's upbringing and appearance; setting up the hammock on the lawn; teasing the cat; talking about politics; and so on.

In this situation care-givers often feel sad and long for a return to "the way it used to be." They feel the loss of security, a sense of certainty, a comfortable feeling of complacency, and familiar family events. They experience the regret of no longer being able to enjoy many shared activities with the care-receiver and of no longer being able to watch a spouse or relative interact with others like he or she used to.

What can you do about it? Knowing that there will be times when you feel miserable and angry that things are the way they are, arrange to spend these times with a friend or do something that will help you over the occasional feeling of helplessness and depression. First, admit that it is normal to feel sad about your situation; second, do something that enables you to express yourself or work out your feelings enough that you can resume your care-giving refreshed, knowing that you are doing what you want to do and have sufficient energy to do it with enthusiasm. Then you can continue to give the care-receiver companionship appropriate for today and tomorrow.

Anticipatory grief is a kind of small mourning that you may go through before your relative dies. For instance, if you decide that you must have help and the care-receiver resents this and becomes distant or rude, you will experience a sense of loss. When you do get help, you may feel that there is something missing in your life — and then realize that you miss the presence of the care-receiver, you miss doing his or her washing (even though you didn't like doing it you still miss it), and so on.

You may also have thought about what it will be like when you spouse or relative is dead. Having such thoughts may make you feel guilty or uneasy. Many of us have been brought up to believe that if you think about something negative or awful it might happen, for example, "Don't write a will or you might die," "Don't think of a person being dead or he might die sooner." This is nonsense. Considering future possibilities is realistic and practical. Thinking about how you will manage and what your life will be like without your relative is planning.

One care-giver whose husband was very ill made arrangements to do volunteer work after her husband died. "It was not easy to do," she recalled. "I was told by several agency workers that I shouldn't be making these plans as my husband would probably get better, and that I was being premature in thinking he would die in a few months. He did die a few months later and it was right (for me) to have decided to arrange something that I could look forward to doing — what I call meaningful activity."

There are counselling and support groups for people who have suffered the loss of someone they love. See Appendix 4 for more on coping with the loss of a loved one.

l. TERMINAL ILLNESS — A LIFE-THREATENING DISORDER

What should you do when the doctor says, "There is nothing more we can do"?

Look at printed material in libraries and in bookstores on the subject of "hospice."

Talk to health department staff in your area — the nurses and social workers in the health units will know what is available in your community that can help you to help your relative or spouse. They can direct you to services that have been set up especially for people who have been told, "There is nothing more we can do." Although there may be no cure at present or in the near future for the disorder your relative has, there are all kinds of things that can be done to keep him or her comfortable.

Appendix 1 at the back of this book has a list of helpful publications dealing with specific disorders and aging; Appendix 2 lists organizations that offer support and information. If your care-receiver has AIDS/HIV, see Appendix 5. These are all places to start in your search for information and support.

m. INDICATORS REQUIRING IMMEDIATE ASSESSMENT

The following signs may indicate that your relative needs help you cannot fully provide. If the care-receiver —

- flinches when you approach;

- is bruised;
- has very red or very white areas or has sores on buttocks and pressure areas such as elbows, back, shoulders, feet or ankles;
- will not cooperate with you but does with others;
- lies to others about what you do or don't do; or
- tells people that you don't love or don't care for him or her,

you should consider turning over the responsibility for care-giving to another.

You should rethink your involvement if —

- others are criticizing what you do or don't do for your relative and this upsets you so that you feel you are always being tested and you fear making decisions that others might criticize;
- you find that you are getting angry and irritable with your relative, family, and friends;
- your main topic of conversation is complaining about your relative; or
- the care-receiver or others criticize your management of the care-receiver's financial affairs.

Reassessing the entire situation and your involvement in it should preferably be done during two or three days away from your relative while you're having a change and a rest.

If you are in doubt about whether the care-receiver is obtaining the basic care needed — physical, social, emotional, and environmental (or, in other words, *food, shelter, clothing, people contact,* and *adequate protection* from injury, infection, and harassment in any form) check with someone you respect such as a minister, community nurse, social worker, doctor or lawyer.

n. LOSS OF ENTHUSIASM

There is a bounce in the step of an enthusiastic person. The healthy individual has an agility, brightness, quick smile, readiness to laugh, and "energy to go" that the ill or frail person does not have.

Guard against losing your enthusiasm for living by making sure that you do not slow down your actions, thinking, and interests in the community as your care-receiver may be doing. Acting sick is not healthy. For example, walking slowly as though you were helping a disabled person cross the street should not become your normal manner of walking if you do not have a mobility problem. If you usually walk quickly, you should continue to do so when you are not guiding a slower person.

Meal planning can become a problem if you don't continue to recognize that you are not the sick person; you can eat what you want. The person on a special diet must get accustomed to seeing you eat normally. If you begin to eat only what your care-receiver eats and at the times he or she eats, convincing yourself that it is easier to make only one menu, you are failing to let the care-receiver face the reality that the household does not revolve around him or her. The other family members are not ill and should not have to act as though they were. Your relative is a part of the household and can enjoy the variation of activities, sights, sounds, and aromas in the home.

One of the excuses care-givers give when challenged by friends who notice that they are beginning to live the lifestyle of the care-receiver is, "But it will make him feel badly since I know he can't eat cheese." Most relatives would be pleased to know that their care-giver is eating foods he or she likes. After all, the care-giver is not the one with the medical problem.

If your care-receiver tends to be unrealistic or unfeeling in this matter, it is up to you to educate him or her or have another person help you do it. The care-receiver should not make your life intolerable by forcing you by words and complaints to live as he or she must. You must preserve your individuality to the point of deliberately having some activities apart from the care-receiver's. This may mean getting help in your home even if the care-receiver becomes a little piqued and jealous.

Remember, you do not have the disorder that limits the care-receiver's activities. You have chosen to help improve the quality of his or her life by assisting where you can, but you are not going to give up everything to do this.

The following signs may indicate that you are losing your enthusiasm and alert you to take steps to get to back what is normal for you:

- decreased speed of walking,
- slower rate of talking,
- slower rate of thinking, reacting and responding,
- decreasing your activities because the care-receiver's activities have decreased,

- slower movements while doing dishes, heavy gardening, getting groceries,
- mimicking the care-receiver's mannerisms, consciously or unconsciously,
- losing interest in the news either on TV or radio or in newspapers,
- losing interest in friends' conversations and activities,
- avoiding activities solely for enjoyment or postponing them indefinitely.

o. LONELINESS

Loneliness is the desperate feeling of wanting to be with one or more companionable people, but being alone.

A lonely person does not need to be so. You can stop being lonely and loneliness can certainly be prevented. To begin with, make sure you are using the right word — that you truly mean lonely and not bored, alone, sad, disappointed, afraid of something like criticism/falling/using incorrect grammar, uncomfortable with some people, embarrassed or shy.

There are five main causes of loneliness:

(a) No money — so little that you don't go anywhere or do anything that you don't consider essential.

(b) No adequate public transportation near you. If you don't want to drive or can't take a taxi, you are dependent on friends and acquaintances. You may eventually not call on them or they may not be available when you wish to go out.

(c) Shut in due to medically diagnosed disability. You stay home because your mobility is severely limited.

(d) Lack of skills and/or knowledge to deal with some situations.

(e) Personality and behavior.

The lonely person is the only one who can overcome the problem. Others can only show a lonely person what is available in the neighborhood or community. The lonely person must then choose to be interested, find out more information, and participate in community events.

We can assist people to overcome their loneliness if it is due to limited income, lack of adequate public transportation, or if they are shut in due to a medical disability — we can help people financially, arrange transportation, and visit shut-ins, bringing with us activities and information from the community.

However, when loneliness is caused by lack of skills and knowledge or by personality and behavior, only the lonely person can learn new skills and acquire knowledge by taking courses, reading, and obtaining counselling. If the lonely person's personality and behavior are not appreciated by others or are such that they interfere with making and keeping friends, only the lonely person can change his or her own personality and behavior. Lonely people must recognize that they are responsible for their own loneliness and that if loneliness is not wanted it can be stopped.

Lonely people can learn skills they have forgotten, such as socializing, exercising, shopping, studying, working, or relaxing.

We as helpers can make opportunities for information and participation available but only the lonely person can create a cure. The best that care-givers can do is to expose the lonely person to all the opportunities they can think of.

p. BURIAL/CREMATION PLANS AND THE WILL

Your care-receiver and other relatives may have questions about arranging a funeral or having a will prepared.

Many care-receivers have neither a will nor burial plans. There is no law that says a person must have a will or make his or her own burial plans. It is true that many relatives and financial advisers suggest that it would certainly be in the best interest of the care-giver and other survivors if there were a will and some indication of funeral arrangements. However, unless the care-receiver asks for the care-giver's opinion on these topics, it is no one's business but the care-receiver's while he or she is alive.

All countries have provisions in law regarding dying intestate (without a will). The estate is usually distributed to immediate next of kin and spouse...eventually.

The family usually makes the funeral plans whether there is a will or not and whether there are burial instructions or not.

1. Burial/cremation plans

A statement in writing of preferences regarding funeral and burial arrangements saves the family and relatives from the uneasiness of speculating on what the care-giver's wishes might have been. This written preference guide alleviates many of the worries about "what should be done" and "what's right," since you know what the care-receiver wants done or does not want done.

If the care-receiver is willing, he or she can write preferences on a sheet of paper or fill out and sign the form included in this book. (See Worksheet #12.)

Someone in the family should know where this information is kept. This way the executor and family can follow the wishes as long as the estate can pay for them and if the instructions are such that most of the family would approve.

Consider the following ABCs of arranging a funeral:

A is for *ashes*. Funeral directors may use the term *cremated remains*.

A is for *attitudes* toward the disposal of the body. If the care-receiver belonged to a religious organization that has specific beliefs, don't make funeral arrangements or disposal arrangements that are contrary to what the church would like. If you are in doubt, check with the minister or priest.

B is for *bereavement*. One of the reasons for putting preferences down on a piece of paper is that bereavement is a very stressful stage of one's life — especially for a spouse, partner, or close next-of-kin. (When I say close, I mean child, father, or mother.) Loss of a spouse is considered the biggest change and largest stress on a person in his or her lifetime. Dr. Thomas Holmes used a scale in which he outlined and assigned points for changes in one's life. The number of points is an indicator of the level of stress in your life. He gave the most points to the loss of a spouse.

One of the reasons for writing down preferences is so the spouse doesn't have extra decisions to make when he or she is already going through a stressful period of his or her life.

C is for *casket*. A firm container is required for every disposal whether for a cremation or for a body burial. The container can be an inexpensive pressed board box. This is a container that funeral homes don't usually put on view. It is usually considered for cremation only. The next cheapest would be a cloth-covered wood box with a flat lid, minimum number of handles, and in a bland color. Casket prices go according to the number of handles, the height of the dome-shaped lid, the material of casket (ranging from cloth-covered wood, to hard wood, to metal) and the ornateness of the handles and the frilliness of the lining.

C is for *cash advance terms*. These are the goods and services that the funeral director purchases on your behalf and then bills you for. Don't assume that you get these for nothing.

C is for *cemetery*. When a body (not ashes) is to be interred, you have to have a plot or grave site. You have to pay to have the grave hole dug and filled in. This is called "opening and closing." There will be extra charges for a marker and for its installation.

C is for *clergy*. If you attend a church and have a minister, priest, or rabbi, he or she should be notified as soon as someone is very ill to be consulted before you make funeral arrangements.

D is for *disposition of the body*. The body can be disposed of in many ways. The cheapest way is to have someone else dispose of it for you and pay for it (e.g., a medical school). That would be the cheapest, but that isn't always what you want and it may not be practical. There are two main ways to dispose of a body: ground burial or cremation. Ashes may be scattered or buried.

D is for *donation* of human parts. Many people would like to give their eyes and kidneys to medicine. The family and the appropriate organizations should know so they can proceed with the arrangements that are necessary when a person dies.

E is for *embalming*. If you don't want embalming, you are going to have to say so because the funeral director routinely embalms, at your expense.

E is for *executor* who can veto any plans previously made. Any unreasonable or overly expensive requests will not be carried out.

F is for *flowers*. Flowers can be specified in the funeral instructions of the deceased. Alternatively, money may be sent to a charity.

F is for *funeral service*. This means a service usually of a religious nature conducted with the body present in an open or closed casket.

G is for *grave* which can be purchased before or after the death. It is considered a piece of real estate.

G is for *grave liner*. This is what the cemeteries have come up with to fill in the slight depression that occurs due to ground settling after the body has been put in a grave. Instead of having an employee refill and reseed or returf a depressed area, grave liners prevent the whole thing happening at all by putting concrete slabs on the sides and top of a casket. This also means you are making another purchase. You might want to look around for a cemetery that doesn't require that you buy a grave liner.

I is for *indigent*. This is someone who has no money. Someone who is indigent and has no burial or funeral instructions will be given a religious service and burial whether it was his or her wish or not. Anyone who is not religious or has very definite ideas on the subject should write them down and let someone know about them.

I is for *item pricing,* which is a method of telling you how much the various goods and services cost that are provided by a funeral director, cemetery, or crematorium. Not many funeral directors use this method although there is a trend toward it. You'll find both types, package deal and item pricing. The better deal may not be much for price, necessarily, but knowing exactly what you are paying for.

L is for *last post fund*. This is an organization that will help with funeral arrangements for veterans who have no money and are not entitled to other veterans' benefits.

M is for *medical schools* that require an almost perfect body. Anyone who plans to donate his or her body to a medical school should make alternate plans because they may not accept you. We've heard elderly people say, "Oh, but I'm so interesting because I've had so many operations. I'm sure they'll take me and besides they've accepted me. I have a paper." That acceptance is only of the application — not the body. If the body suits the requirements after death, that is when the body may be accepted.

M is for *memorial service*. This means a service, a eulogy, in memory of the deceased but the body is not present. A memorial service is sometimes less formal than a funeral service.

M is for *memorial societies*. These are organizations that make arrangements for members. They give their members an opportunity for certain types of arrangements and attempt, after the member dies, to see that the arrangements he or she chose are carried out with the approval of the executor and next-of-kin.

N is for *notice* — death notice or instructions regarding the various towns or cities where death notices should be placed in newspapers. These notices don't cost that much compared to the comfort it will give survivors to receive sympathy letters and cards from distant relatives and old friends.

O is for *official administrator*. If a person dies without a will, the official administrator will be asked to look after the estate. There is no law that requires a person to have a will, but it has been proven time and again that it is better for the survivors if there is one.

P is for *post-funeral reception*. This is a gathering of family and friends after the funeral.

R is for *reasonably priced*. Reasonably — meaning what? This is what you must find out. The expression is sometimes used in funeral directors' advertising.

S is for the *safety deposit box* where burial and funeral instructions should not be kept because usually the contents are looked at after the disposal of the body and the service.

S is for *services*. Normally, when you think of services in connection with funerals and burials you think of a funeral service or memorial service or graveside service. But that is not what a funeral director or cemetery administrator means. The word "services" in advertising by the funeral industry can mean anything in the way of goods or services that the industry may offer you.

T is for *transporting* the body. Sometimes a body is buried in another country, perhaps where the person was born. Cost is the biggest factor. If a person has the money and the executor does not feel that the preference is unreasonable then that is what will be done.

U is for *urns*. Cremation is not very expensive, but if you buy an expensive urn and an expensive plot and marker, it can add up. Cremation is only cheaper if you keep all costs down.

V is for *viewing* the body. Unless specified, a body will normally be viewed.

W is for *wake* which we really don't have now. In some places perhaps viewing the body and serving coffee and cookies at the funeral home can be considered a modern version.

If your care-receiver has wishes or preferences on how he or she wants to be buried, consider using Worksheet #12.

2. The will

Your care-receiver may want your assistance in drawing up his or her will. Here are some pointers on how you can help.

(a) Call a notary or a lawyer and make an appointment.

(b) Obtain a form will from your local stationery store (also available from the publisher) so you know what basic information you need to make even the simplest will. Use it as a learning tool to familiarize yourself with the vocabulary.

(c) Help the care-receiver fill out the form in pencil and make any necessary notes.

WORKSHEET #12
BURIAL PLANS

Instructions in the Event of My Death

When I'm dead I would like my family and executor(s) to comply with my preferences for my burial to the best of their ability.

I Plans made

I have made funeral and burial arrangements with_____
_____
Funeral Home/society/association. See the attached papers or locate them_____
and/or _____

I have arranged to donate my (body or parts of body)_____
_____ to _____
See the attached information or locate papers at _____.

II My body

As I have not made arrangements with a funeral home or burial society, I choose to indicate my preferences as marked.

1. I choose to be buried.   Yes ____ No ____
   - (a) As soon as possible, no service being held _____
     Before service _____
     After service _____
   - (b) To be embalmed   Yes ____ No ____
   - (c) To be viewed   Yes ____ No ____
   - (d) Type of casket:_____
   - (e) Cemetery name and location:_____
     _____
     or
     Mausoleum name and location: _____
     _____
   - (f) Comments: _____
     _____

2. I choose to be cremated   Yes ____ No ____
   - (a) As soon as possible, no service being held _____
     Before service _____
     After service _____

WORKSHEET #12 — Continued

    (b) Prior to cremation:
        (1) To be embalmed   Yes ____ No ____
        (2) To be viewed   Yes ____ No ____
        (3) Type of container or casket: _____
    (c) I choose that my cremated remains (ashes):
        Be scattered _____ Be buried _____ Be placed _____
        I have no particular preferences _____
    (d) Location for cremated remains (ashes) — cemetery, mausoleum or other designated place:
        _____
    (e) Comments: _____
        _____

3. More considerations
    Urn   Yes ____ No ____ Comments:_____
    Grave liner Yes ____ No ____ Comments: _____
    Gravestone Yes ____ No ____ Comments: _____
    Monument   Yes ____ No ____ Comments: _____
    Marker   Yes ____ No ____ Comments:_____
    Flowers   Yes ____ No ____ Comments:_____
    Other preferences: _____

III Gatherings
- I do not want a service _____
- I do not want a reception _____
- I would like family and friends to gather after I am dead. I am aware that the cost for a service and/or reception will come from my estate. _____

1. Service
    (a) Type
        Funeral service (body present)_____
        Memorial service (body not present)_____
        Graveside service_____
    (b) Minister, priest or speaker   Yes _____ No _____

WORKSHEET #12 — Continued

        If yes, state name of person preferred:
        _____
- (c) Place of service (name and address): _____
  _____
- (d) Transportation for family   Yes _____   No_____
- (e) Procession to cemetery   Yes _____   No_____
- (f) Flowers   Yes _____   No_____
- (g) Music   Yes _____   No_____
- (h) Death notice in newspaper   Yes _____   No_____
  (If yes, see details in section **IV**)
- (i) List of names of people at the service   Yes _____   No_____
- (j) Comments: _____

2. Reception
   - If yes, state location:
   - Family residence
   - Relative or friend's home (name and address): _____
     _____
   - Public place, e.g., restaurant or rented hall _____
   - Other premises _____
   - I would like also: _____

IV Death notices

1. If friends and family want to donate or do something in memory of me, I'd like them to:

    Send flowers to chapel, family and/or gravesite _____
    Send Mass cards _____
    Other_____
    I have no strong feelings in this matter _____

2. If my preferences are complied with, it is my wish that the death notice in the papers states: "Arrangements as requested by the deceased."   Yes_____   No _____

3. I'd like a notice placed in the following newspapers:
    Local: _____   Out-of-town: _____

WORKSHEET #12 — Continued

4. Where I used to live: _____

Please put in a few words besides the essentials, for instance:
- member of _____
- formerly of (city, country) _____
- recently from _____
- was employee of _____ company for _____ years
- served with _____
- was a volunteer with _____ association/organization
- was founder of _____
- after retirement continued to follow/support/maintain interest in _____
- for many years maintained interest in _____
- enthusiastic/regular supporter of _____
- organization/association _____

I am aware that the cost of death notice(s) will be paid from my estate.

OTHER:

Signature_____
Name in full _____
Date _____

(d) A directives list should be made — a list of the things the care-receiver would like the executor to do that there is no place for on the form will.

(e) A lot of time and money can be saved if these preparations are made before visiting a notary or lawyer.

I suggest that you consider making a beneficiary executor as beneficiaries have the most to gain in settling the estate properly.

The executor is free to hire a trust company or lawyer or notary to help carry out the duties should the need arise. I do not recommend that a financial institution or lawyer be named in the will unless your beneficiaries are minors or incompetent (in the legal sense). The advisers named may not be appropriate by the time of the death. It is better, in my opinion, to put the choices of legal and financial consultants in the directives to the executor, which are not legally binding. This provides the executor the freedom to choose his or her own technical and expert advice should it be required.

The age of your executor is unimportant as long as he or she is a legal adult. Even if the named executor is younger than the person writing the will, there is no assurance that the person will live longer. If the executor becomes ill, unfriendly, irrational, or inadequate in any way, another should be appointed by adding a codicil to the will.

A lawyer will want all belongings that have real monetary value listed in your will. However, if a person doesn't want all his or her possessions sold and the money divided up, he or she can write a directive to the executor asking that the articles be distributed among the beneficiaries.

The directive is only a guide to the executor; the executor does not have to comply with it as he or she must comply with the instructions in the will. The directive is an excellent way to plan the distribution of sentimental and personal items in the estate. Items to consider for a directive list include household belongings, clothes, plants, pets, pictures, paintings, lamps, dishes, furniture, costume jewelry, luggage, collections (salt and pepper shakers, match boxes, dolls, comic books, jugs, cookbooks, etc.), books, records (music), family history records, and photos. An example of a directives list is shown in Sample #4.

SAMPLE #4
DIRECTIVES LIST

Directives

Jane	*Elizabeth*	*Arthur*
piano	bone china cups and saucers	tools (workshop and gardening)
family photos	sewing machine	grandfather clock
linen	dishwasher (portable)	pocket watch
china tea service	fur coat	beer mugs and bar tools and supplies

APPENDIX 1
HELPFUL PUBLICATIONS

a. GENERAL

Buzan, Tony. *Use Both Sides of Your Brain*. Plume Books: New York, 1986.

Hanson, Peter G. *Counterattack: The Joy of Stress Action Plan for Gaining Control of Your Life and Health*. Stoddart Publishing: Toronto, 1993.

The 12 Steps for Adult Children (from addictive and other dysfunctional families). (Revised ed.) Recovery Publications, Inc: San Diego, CA, 1989.

Woititz, Janet M. and Alan Garner. *Lifeskills for Adult Children*. Health Communications Inc.: Deerfield, Florida, 1990.

b. SPECIFIC DISORDERS

Alcoholics Anonymous. (3rd Edition). Alcoholics Anonymous, New York, 1976.

Bartlett, John G. and Ann K. Kinkbeiner. *The Guide to Living with HIV Infection*. (Revised ed.) Johns Hopkins University Press, 1993.

Carroll, David L. *Living with Parkinson's*. HarperCollins Publishers: New York, 1992.

Cavel-Grant, Deborah. *You, Me and Myasthenia Gravis*. Available from the author: 514 — 4637 McLeod Trail, Calgary, Alberta T2G 5C1. 1993.

Eidson, Ted, ed. *The AIDS Caregiver's Handbook*. St. Martin's Press: New York, 1988.

Ellert, Gwen and John Wade. *The Osteoporosis Book*. Trelle Enterprises Inc.: Vancouver, 1993.

Goldenbery, S. Larry. *Prostate Cancer*. Intelligent Patient Guide: Vancouver, 1992.

Horner, Pamela. *Osteoporosis: The Long Road Back*. University of Ottawa Press: Ottawa, 1989.

Jacobowitz, Ruth S. *150 Most-asked Questions about Osteoporosis*. Hearst Books: New York, 1993.

Kowalski, Robert E. *8 Steps to a Healthy Heart*. Warner Books: New York, 1992.

Krohn, Jaqueline, et al. *The Whole Way to Allergy Relief Prevention*. Hartley and Marks Inc.: Vancouver, 1991.

Lieberman, Abraham N. and Frank L. Williams. *Parkinson's Disease: The complete guide for patients and caregivers*. Fireside Books: New York, 1993.

Mace, Nancy L. and Peter V. Raabins. *The 36-Hour Day: A family guide to caring for persons with Alzheimer's disease, related dementing illnesses, and memory loss in later life*. Warner Books: New York, 1984.

Martelli, Leonard J. with Fran D. Peltz and William Messina. *When Someone You Know Has AIDS: A practical guide*. (Revised ed.) Crown Publishers: New York, 1993.

Matthews, Bryan. *Multiple Sclerosis: The Facts*. Oxford University Press: Toronto, 1993.

McIlwain, Harris H. et al. *Winning with Osteoporosis*. John Wiley and Sons Inc.: New York, 1993.

Narcotic Anonymous N.A. World Service Office, Inc. Van Nuys, CA Fifth editon: 1988.

Nessim, Susan and Judith Ellis. *Cancervive: The Challenge of Life after Cancer*. Houghton Mifflin Company: New York, 1991.

Schapiro, Randall T. *Symptom Management in Multiple Sclerosis*. Demos Publications: New York, 1993.

Scheinberg, Labe (Ed.). *Multiple Sclerosis: A guide for patients and their families*. (2nd ed.) Raven Press: New York, 1987.

Simmerman, Barry, et al. *The Canadian Allergy & Asthma Handbook*. Random House: Toronto, 1991.

Vancouver Persons with AIDS Society. *Positive Living: A manual for people affected by AIDS/HIV*. (Revised ed.) Vancouver Persons with AIDS Society, 1107 Seymour Street, Vancouver, B.C., Canada V6B 5S8, 1993.

Whitehead, Mark and Brent Patterson. *Managing Your Health: A guide for people living with HIV or AIDS*. Community AIDS Treatment Information Exchange (CATIE) and The Toronto People with AIDS Foundation, 1993.

Wood, Lawrence C., et. al. *Your Thyroid*. Ballantine Books: New York, 1982.

b. AGING

Manning, Doug. *Socks — How to Solve Problems*. In-Sight Books, Inc.: Texas, 1989.

Edinberg, Mark A. *Talking with your aging Parents*. Shambhala: Boston, 1988.

Chapman, Elwood N. *The Unfinished Business of Living: Helping aging parents help themselves*. Crisp Publications, Inc.: Los Altos, California, 1988.

c. DYING AND DEATH

Buckman, Robert. *I don't know what to say: How to help and support someone who is dying*. Key Porter Books: Toronto, 1988.

Campbell, Scott and Phyllis Silverman. *The Widower*. Prentice Hall Inc.: New York, 1987.

Diets, Bob M. *Life after Loss: A personal guide dealing with death, divorce, job change, and relocation*. Fisher Books: Tucson, Arizona, 1988.

Di Guilio, Robert C. *Beyond Widowhood*. Free Press: New York, 1989.

Palmer, Elsie and Jill Watt. *Living and Working with Bereavement: Guide for widowed men and women*. Detselig Enterprises Ltd.: Calgary, 1987.

Rando, Therese A. *Grieving: How to go on living when someone you love dies*. Lexington Books: Mass., 1988.

Staudacher, Carol. *Men and Grief*. New Harbinger Publications Inc.: Oakland, CA, 1991.

Tatelbaum, Judy. *The Courage to Grieve: Creative living, recovery and growth through grief*. Lippincott and Crowell, HarperCollins Publishers: New York, 1984.

APPENDIX 2
ADDRESSES

Here is a list of associations in the United States and Canada and overseas that you may find useful.

To contact an association, write saying, "Please send me information on your organization. Do you have a branch in our area?" Be sure to include your name and return address. Print your name under your signature (in case they can't read it). Allow three weeks for a reply. You will be pleased with the informational brochures you receive.

If you have more questions, write to them again or talk to your public health nurse or family doctor and check out your local library.

If you are not currently a family care-giver but are interested in the subject of, say, heart disease, you can still write to the Heart Foundation for information of a general nature. However, specific information regarding your own or your relative's health will only be given to you by your physician.

a. CANADA

Alcoholics Anonymous, Toronto (AA)
#502, 234 Eglinton Avenue E.
Toronto, Ontario
M4P 1K5
(416) 487-5591

Allergy Asthma Information Association (AAIA)
#10, 65 Tromley Drive
Islington, Ontario
M9B 5Y7
(905) 244-9312

Alzheimer Society of Canada
#201, 1320 Yonge Street
Toronto, Ontario
M4T 1X2
(416) 925-3552

Amyotrophic Lateral Sclerosis Society of Canada (ALS)
#B101, 90 Adelaide Street E.
Toronto, Ontario
M5C 2R4
(416) 362-0269

The Arthritis Society
#401, 250 Bloor Street E.
Toronto, Ontario
M4W 1E6
(416) 967-1414

Asthma Society of Canada
P.O.Box 213, Stn. K
Toronto, Ontario
(416) 977-9684

Canadian Aids Society (CAS)
701 - 100, rue Sparks Street
Ottawa, Ontario
K1P 5B7
(613) 230-3580

Canadian Association of Friedreich's Ataxia (ACAF)
5620, rue C.A. Jobin
Montreal, Quebec H1P 1H8

Canadian Cancer Society
#200, 10 Alcorn Avenue
Toronto, Ontario
M4V 3B1
(416) 961-7223

Canadian Celiac Association
6519 B Mississauga Road
Mississauga, Ontario
L5N 1A6
(905) 567-7195

Canadian Cerebral Palsy Association
City Centre
#612, 880 Wellington
Ottawa, Ontario
K1R 6K7
1-800-267-6572

Canadian Diabetes Association
78 Bond Street
Toronto, Ontario
M5B 2J8
(416) 362-4440

Canadian Down's Syndrome Society
#206, 12837 76th Avenue
Surrey, B.C.
V3W 2V3
(604) 599-6009

Canadian Hearing Society
271 Spadina Road
Toronto, Ontario
M5R 2V3
(416) 964-9595

Canadian Lung Association
#908, 75 Albert Street
Ottawa, Ontario
K1H 5E7
(613) 237-1208

Canadian Mental Health Association (CMHA)
3rd Floor, 2160 Yonge Street
Toronto, Ontario
M4S 2Z3
(416) 484-7750

Canadian National Institute for the Blind (CNIB)
1931 Bayview Avenue
Toronto, Ontario
M4G 4C8
(416) 480-7580

The Canadian Red Cross Society
1800 Alta Vista Drive
Ottawa, Ontario
K1G 4J5
(613) 739-2217

Canadian Stroke Recovery Association
#122A, 170 The Donway W.
Don Mills, Ontario
M3C 2G3
(905) 441-1421

Epilepsy Canada
#745, 470 Peel Street
Montreal, Quebec
H3A 1T1
(514) 845-7855

Heart and Stroke Foundation of Canada
#200 - 160 George Street
Ottawa, Ontario
K1N 9M2
(613) 237-4361

Huntington Society of Canada
3 - 13 Water Street N.
P.O. Box 333
Cambridge, Ontario
N1R 5T8
(519) 622-1002

Lupus Canada (1989)
P.O. Box 3302, Stn. B.
Calgary, Alberta
T2M 4L8
1-800-661-1468

Multiple Sclerosis Society of Canada
#820, 250 Bloor Street E.
Toronto, Ontario
M4W 3P9
(416) 922-6065

Muscular Dystrophy Association of Canada
#400, 150 Eglinton Avenue E.
Toronto, Ontario
M4P 1E8
(416) 488-0030

Myasthenia Gravis Association of British Columbia
2805 Kingsway
Vancouver, B.C.
V5R 5H9
(604) 451-5511

Narcotics Anonymous
P.O. Box 5700
Toronto, Ontario
M5W 1N8
(416) 498-6148

Osteoporosis Society of Canada
33 Laird Drive
Toronto, Ontario
M4G 3S9
(416) 696-2663

Parkinson Foundation of Canada
#232, 55 Bloor Street W.
Toronto, Ontario
M4W 1A6
(416) 251-8141

St. John Ambulance
312 Laurier Avenue E.
P.O. Box 388, Stn. A
Ottawa, Ontario
K1N 8V4
(613) 236-7461

Tourette Syndrome Foundation of Canada
238 Davenport Road
P.O. Box 343
Toronto, Ontario
M5R 1J6
(416) 968-2009

United Ostomy Association Canada
P15, 296 Mill Road
Etobicoke, Ontario
M9C 4X8
(416) 626-5981

World Federation of Hemophilia (WFH)
4616 Street Catherine Street W.
Montreal, Quebec
H3Z 1S3

b. UNITED STATES

Alcoholics Anonymous
11th Floor, 475 Riverside Drive
New York, NY 10115
(212) 870-3400

Alcoholics Anonymous World Services (AA)
P.O. Box 459
Grand Central Station
New York, NY 10163
(212) 686-1000

ALS and Neuromuscular Research Foundation (ALSNRF)
c/o Pacific Presbyterian Center
No. 416, 2351 Clay Street
San Francisco, CA 94115
(415) 923-3604

Alzheimer's Disease and Related Disorders Association, Inc.
Suite 1000, 919 N. Michigan Avenue
Chicago, IL 60600-1676
(312) 335-8700

American Cancer Society (ACS)
1599 Clifton Road N.E.
Atlanta, GA 30329
800-ACS-2345

American Council of the Blind
Suite 720, 1155 15th Street N.W.
Washington, DC 20005
(202) 467-5081

American Diabetes Association
1660 Duke Street
Alexandria, VA 22314
(703) 549-1500

American Heart Association
7272 Greenville Avenue
Dallas, TX 75231-4596
(214) 373-6300

American Lung Association
1740 Broadway
New York, NY 10019-4374
(212) 315-8700

American Red Cross
17th and D Sts. N.W.
Washington, DC 20006
(202) 737-8300

Amyotrophic Lateral Sclerosis Association (ALSA)
Ste. 321, 21021 Ventura Boulevard
Woodland Hills, CA 91364
(818) 340-7500

Arthritis Foundation
1314 Spring Street N.W.
Atlanta, GA 30309
(404) 872-7100

CDC National AIDS Clearinghouse
U.S. Department of Health and Human Services
P.O. Box 6003
Rockville, MD 20849-6003
1-800-458-5231

Dystonia Medical Research Foundation (DMRF)
No. 800, 8383 Wilshire Blvd.
Beverly Hills, CA 90211
(213) 852-1630

Eldercare Locator
800-677-1116

Epilepsy Concern Service Group (EC)
1282 Wynnewood Drive
West Palm Beach, FL 33417
(407) 683-0044

Epilepsy Foundation of America (EFA)
4351 Garden City Drive
Landover, MD 20785
(301) 459-3700

Family Caregiver Alliance Association
Suite 500
425 Bush Street
San Francisco, CA 94108
(415) 434-3388

Friedreich's Ataxia Group in America (FAGA)
P.O. Box 11116
Oakland, CA 94611-0116
(415) 655-0833

Huntington's Disease Society of America (HDSA)
6th Floor, 140 W. 22nd Street
New York, NY 10011-2420
(212) 242-1968

Lupus Foundation of America, Inc.
Suite 180
4 Research Place
Rockville, MD 20850-3226
1-800-3226 and (301) 670-9292

Myasthenia Gravis Foundation (MG)
Ste. 1352, 53 W. Jackson Blvd.
Chicago, IL 60604
(312) 427-6252

Muscular Dystrophy
3300 E. Sunrise Drive
Tuscon, AZ 85718
(602) 529-2000

Narcotics Anonymous (NA)
P.O. Box 9999
Van Nuys, CA 91409
(818) 780-3951

National Association of the Deaf
814 Thayer Avenue
Silver Spring, MD 20910
(301) 587-1788

National Family Caregivers Association
9223 Longbranch Parkway
Silver Spring, MD 20901-3642
(301) 949-3638

National Federation of the Blind
1800 Johnson Street
Baltimore, MD 21230
(410) 659-9314

National Head Injury Foundation (NHIF)
333 Turnpike Road
Southborough, MA 01772
(508) 485-9950

National Mental Health Association
1021 Prince Street
Alexandria, VA 22314-2971
(703) 684-7722

National Multiple Sclerosis Society
733 Third Avenue
New York, NY 10017-3288
(212) 986-3240

National Parkinson Foundation (NPF)
1501 N.W. 9th Avenue
Miami, FL 33136
(305) 547-6666

National Spinal Cord Injury Association (NSCIA)
Ste. 2000, 600 W. Cummings Park
Woburn, MA 01801
(617) 935-2722

National Stroke Association (NSA)
Ste. 240, 300 E. Hampden Avenue
Englewood, CO 80110
(303) 762-9922

Parkinson Support Groups of America (PSGA)
No. 204, 11376 Cherry Hill Road
Bettsville, MD 20705
(301) 937-1545

Parkinson's Educational Program — U.S.A. ((PEP/USA)
No. 105, 3900 Birch Street
Newport Beach, CA 92660
(714) 250-2975

Stroke Clubs
International (SCI)
805 12th Street, Galveston, TX 77550
(409) 762-1022

Tourette Syndrome Association (TSA)
42-40 Bell Boulevard
Bayside, NY 11361
(718) 224-2999

United Parkinson Foundation (UPF)
360 W. Superior Street
Chicago, IL 60610
(312) 664-2344

c. AUSTRALIA

Aged Care Australia
P.O. Box 303
Curtin ACT 2605
(06) 285 3097

Aged Services Association of NSW and ACT Inc.
Suite 1, Murray Arcade
127-133 Burwood Road
Burwood, NSW 2134
(02) 745 2999

Alcohol and Drug Foundation
Victoria, P.O. Box 529
153 Park Street South
Melbourne, Victoria 3205
(03) 690 6000

Arthritis Foundation of Australia
Suite 421 Wingello House
Angel Place
Sydney, NSW 2000
(02) 221 2456

Asthma Foundation of New South Wales
Suite 1/82-86 Pacific Highway
Street Leonards NSW 2065
(02) 906 3233

Asthma Foundation of Victoria
2 Highfield Grove
Kew, Viv 3101
(03) 853 5666

Australian Cancer Society Inc.
G.P.O. Box 4708
Sydney NSW 2001
(02) 358 2066

Australian Council on the Aging
3rd floor, VACC House
464 Street Kilda Road
Melbourne, Vic 3004
(03) 820 2655

Australian Council for the Rehabilitation
of the Disabled (ACROD)
Thessiger Court
Deakin, ACT 2600

Australian Deafness Council
P.O. Box 60
Curtin ACT 2605

Australia Federation of
AIDS Organisations Inc. (AFAO)
P.O. Box 525
Woden ACT 2606
616 285 4464

Better Hearing Australia (BHA)
P.O. Box 454
West End, Queensland 4101

Deaf-Blind Care Association
P.O. Box 267
Clifton Hill 3068
600 Nicholson Street
North Fitzroy, Vic 3068
(03) 482 1155

Deafness Foundation
Victoria, Box 42
Nunawading, Vic 3131
(03) 887 8848

Huntington Society
c/o R. Capp
P.O. Box 247
Lidcombe, NSW 2141

National Epilepsy Association of Australia
1st Floor, 184 Main Street
Lilydale, Vic 3140
(03) 735 0211

National Heart Foundation of Australia
P.O. Box 2
Woden ACT 2606
(06) 282 2144

Technical Aid to the Disabled
P.O. Box 108
Ryde, NSW 2112
(02) 808 2022

d. GREAT BRITAIN AND NORTHERN IRELAND

Action Against Allergy (AAA)
24-26 High Street
Hampton Hill, Middx TWl2 1PD

Alcoholics Anonymous
P.O. Box 1
Stonebow House
Stonebow, York
YOI 2NJ
0904-644026

Alzheimer's Disease Society (ADS)
158-160 Balham High Road
London SW12 9BN
081-675 6557

Arthritis Care
18 Stephenson Way
London NWI 2HD
071-916 1500

British Association for Service to the Elderly (BASE)
119 Hassell Street
Newcastle-under-Lyme, Staffs ST5 1AX
0782 661033

British Association of Cancer United Patients
121-123 Charterhouse Street
London ECIM 6AA
071-696 9003

British Diabetic Association
10 Queen Ann Street
London WIM 0BD
071-323 1531

British Red Cross
9 Grosvenor Crescent
London SWIX 7EJ
071-235 5454

British Deaf Association
38 Victoria Race
Carlisle CAI IHU
0228-48844

British Polio Fellowship
Bell Close
West End Road
Ruislip, Middx HA4 6LP
089 567 5515

Carers National Association
29 Chilworth Mews
London W23RG
071 724 7776

Families Anonymous (FA)
310 Finchley Road
London NW3 7AG
071-431 3537

The Federation of Deaf Management Societies
Stede Court
Biddenden
Ashford, Kent TN27 8JG
0580-291235

Friedreich's Ataxia Group (FAX)
Copse Edge
Thursley Road
Elstead, Godalming
Surrey GU8 6DJ

Help the Aged
Street James Walk
Clerkenwell Green
London ECIR OBE
071-253 0253

Huntington's Disease Association (ACHC)
108 Battersea High Street
London SW11 3HP

International Cerebral Palsy Society (ICPS)
5A Netherhall Gardens
London NW3 5RN

International Federation of Multiple Sclerosis Societies (IFMSS)
3/9 Heddon Street
London WIR 7LE

Lupus U.K.
P.O. 999, Romford
Essex RM1 1DW
0708 731251

Mental After Care Association
Bainbridge House
Bainbridge Street
London WCIA 1HP
071 436 6194

The Mental Health Foundation
8 Hallam Street
London WIN 6DH
071-580 0145

Multiple Sclerosis Society
25 Effie Road
London SW6 1EE
071-736 6267

Muscular Dystrophy Group of Great Britain and Northern Ireland
Nattrass House
35 Macauley Road
London SW4 0QP
44-71720 8055

National Association for Colitis and Crohn's Disease (NACC)
98a London Road
Street Albans ALI 1NX
0727 44296

National Listening Library
12 Lant Street
London SEI 1QH
071-407 9417

National Schizophrenia Fellowship
28 Castle Street
Kingston upon Thames
Surrey KTI 1SS
081-547 3937

Parkinson's Disease Society
22 Upper Woburn Place
London WC1H 0RA
071-383 3513

Patients Association
18 Victoria Park Square
London E2 9PF
081-981 5676

The Relative Association
c/o Counsel and Care
Twyman House
16 Bonny Street
London NW1 9PG
071-284-2541 or 081-201-9153

Royal Association in Aid of Deaf People
27 Old Oak Road
London W3 7HN
081-743 6187

Royal National Institute for the Blind (RNIB)
224 Great Portland Street
London WIN 6AA
071-388 1266

Spinal Injuries Association (SIA)
Newpoint House
76 Street James Ln.
London N10 3DF

St. John Ambulance
1 Grosvenor Crescent
London SW1X 7EF
071 235 5231

The Stroke Association
CHSA House
Whitecross Street
London EC1Y 8JJ
071-490 7999

Terrence Higgins Trust (AIDS information)
52-54 Grays Inn Road
London WC1X 8JU
071 831 0330

World Federation for Cancer Care (WFCC)
44 Ladbroke Road
London WII 3NW

e. REPUBLIC OF IRELAND

Irish Cancer Society
5 Northumberland Road
Dublin 4
353 (1) 681855

Irish Deaf Society
Carmichael House
North Brunswick Street
Dublin 7
353 (1) 725748 & 735702

Irish Diabetic Association
82-83 Lower Gardiner Street
Dublin 1
353 (1) 363022

Irish Red Cross
16 Merrion Square
Dublin 2
353 (1) 765135

f. SCOTLAND

Scottish Association for the Deaf (SAD)
Moray House College
Holyrood Road
Edinburgh EH8 8AQ
031-556 0591

Scottish Down's Syndrome Association (SDSA)
158-160 Balgreen Road
Edinburgh EH11 3AU
031-3134225

Scottish Huntington's Association
61 Main Road
Elderslie, PA5 9BA
0505 22245

Scottish Society for the Mentally Handicapped (SSMH)
13 Elmbank Street
Glasgow G2 4QA
041-226 4541

Scottish Spinal Cord Injury Association (SSCIA)
Unit 22, 100 Elderpark Street
Glasgow G51 3TR
041-440 096

APPENDIX 3
RESPONSES TO "RELATIVES CARING FOR RELATIVES" QUESTIONNAIRE

1. When you became the care-giver, was it because of one of the following reasons — duty; you were the oldest; loyalty; closest in age to relative; ill relative liked you best; you wanted to, had the time, knew what to do — or for any other reason?

   Most frequent replies were oldest daughter, live in same town, knew what to do.

2. About how long have you been managing the affairs of your ill relative or friend?

   Most frequent replies were between three months and five years.

3. What are some of the activities you do that especially help you to manage the ill relative's household, nursing, financial, and social affairs?

   Selected responses:
   - obtained legal power of attorney — bank manager helpful
   - close relationship with director of nursing home
   - ask for advice from social worker and lawyer
   - try to carry on as normally as possible
   - spend a lot of time organizing routines
   - schedule hospital visits into my daily routine
   - I found I have to be extremely organized in order to keep my own home and family together while I care for my father
   - hire a nurse for daytime
   - I treat my mother as if she could help me in many ways
   - arrange things by phone
   - have become very single-minded and aggressive to get the care and attention required
   - keep business acquaintances and friends informed

- have learned to be a list-maker — to help me and to help others helping me
- have consolidated my parents' money and moved it to a bank near where I live and got signing authority for myself and my sister
- my sister and I take turns visiting
- arrange for occasional mobile meal service
- an older lady friend helper living in the home relieves me tremendously
- I have cut out all activities. I had a non-listed phone installed — well worth the expense as I would take the listed phone off the hook for hours
- Being away from my home and looking after the patient who lives in an apartment, I quite enjoy the friendship of his neighbors who invite me to teas, lunches, or dinner for an hour's break

4. What are some of your activities that especially help you with your own affairs (emotional and physical health, social and educational activities, and financial concerns)?

Selected responses:
- work full-time during the day
- care for teenage sons, husband, and house
- keep up socially with my husband's and my own friends and play bridge twice a month
- alternate with members of the family to do daily visiting
- get out of the house to pursue my own activities — meetings, courses, lunch or dinner with friends
- ride my horses, try to continue with school
- talk with friends
- two evenings a week to do my own shopping and maintain my home — also work full-time
- the church, friends who call to visit
- teaching, activities related to professional interests, my children and friends
- my sister sent me to a resort for ten days' rest while she took over the nursing

- I started a new sweater so I'd have something to do with my hands while endlessly waiting
- mother took the children for a few months so I could be with my husband
- I write a record of events and my feelings during the year
- sound off to other relatives also looking after ill family member
- plan activities to go to even if I have to cancel at the last minute
- my husband supports me all the way
- church programs, professional educational activities, golf, driving car
- hire a sitter so that we can get out
- entertain friends and get away for short periods
- mission work, satisfying social contacts
- I took up swimming and a refresher course in nursing
- when shopping, I take a little portable radio and on my way back drive by the beach and sit for 10 to 20 minutes, relax, look at the scenery and listen to music
- I make the most of the company that comes to see the invalid and serve tea every time. However, there are many days that I hang a notice on the door, "Sorry, no visitors today," when the invalid is too sick.

5. What tasks or activities do other people do for the ill relative that you find especially helpful?

Selected responses:

- social worker helped choose nursing home — neighbors come in occasionally
- people come to visit; husband takes ill relative (father) out for drives
- hospital arrangements and admittance
- cooking, visiting, feeding, bathing, reading to, just being there
- talking, making suggestions
- visiting her in the nursing home
- social visiting — family member provides vacation relief, which is a life-saver

- call, send letters, phone, give her good food
- a friend, an RN, spent almost all her off-duty time with my mother the last couple of days. People volunteer constantly to do anything and everything
- take care of her dogs and cats
- make telephone calls to friends and relatives for me
- keeping appointments and being on time, visiting, consideration and tolerance for Dad's slowness in walking and answering
- occasional outings and visits. Visitors bring gifts for special occasions. Minister visits regularly
- take them out for a drive or visit, so we have a break
- my brother and his wife, who live out of town, invited her to visit them for as long as she liked — she stayed for three months
- tremendous help to have someone offer their husband as a handyman, who could install a handrail or fix a clothesline, etc., which was beyond my capabilities. One friend lent us a wheelchair which I kept in the car and another wheelchair was in the house

6. What things would you like other people to do to help you?

Selected responses:

- more explanation to patient by doctor. We had to always press for details and no one seemed to give information on changes in condition
- someone to take him for a drive or stay with him while I was out
- people to visit her more often, rather than send plants and flowers that she cannot see and has minimum space for
- acknowledgement of grief, acceptance of feelings, to withhold that trite "everything is going to be all right"
- more assistance (moral, emotional) from family members
- volunteer to stay with Mom for a couple of hours so I could perhaps go out somewhere
- more attention given to the selection and training of nursing home staff
- physiotherapy and occupational therapy programs

- more understanding when I am unable to keep some social engagements and less "why don't you get a babysitter?"
- help me find a less expensive drug store
- professionals calling me instead of me them — and call regularly
- homemaker service that I could afford
- professionals to consider me and my life too and realize that 24-hour-a-day responsibility can get you down after a while
- same professionals — not different ones every month or so — having to say things over, get used to different doctors' ways and names
- report on the patient's condition every so often
- understand the concern I feel and the energy it takes to make decision after decision
- family members spend more time and not leave it mostly to us
- someone to whom I can talk and share some of my difficulties and frustrations
- send notes to the patient rather than phone
- I would like others to keep their distance instead of butting in and making things so difficult for the relative to handle the patient — for his own good
- my sisters to plan a definite day (full day) to take her out so that I knew I could plan on having for myself
- an in-law suite for my mother so we aren't so cramped for space and the children could have more room

APPENDIX 4
DEALING WITH GRIEF*

Grief is the natural reaction you have when someone you love has died. Each person's response to a traumatic loss is unique and often a frightening and confusing experience. The process of grief affects us psychologically, socially, and physically.

a. PSYCHOLOGICAL

Grieving means experiencing many emotions, not just those of sadness and depression. Some emotions you may have had at some time — others will be new and unfamiliar. Many people have the feeling that they will lose control even "go crazy." These are normal feelings during this painful process called grief. Some of the feelings associated with grief are: fearful, anxious, angry, guilty, questioning of your faith, longing for the person, depressed, despairing, sad, confused, less concentration, lapses in memory, less self-esteem, less self concern, emptiness.

It is important to have a family member or friend to talk with at this time and perhaps your doctor or minister or counselor can help you during this long process of grieving.

b. SOCIAL

When a person has a serious loss their social life can be dramatically affected. This usually adds to the sense of confusion and lowering further of your self-esteem. The most common social problems are: restlessness, lack of interest in normal activities, bored with others' conversation and often irritated by them. Your preoccupation with grief may make it difficult to engage in your normal social interactions at work and home. It may also be painful to see people being happy. You may want to be alone often but don't be alone too often. You may also want to keep very busy to avoid the pain of your loss

---

*by Lynette Pollard-Elgert, Executive Director of Living Through Loss Counselling Society, Vancouver, B.C. Reprinted with permission.

but don't keep so busy that you postpone or avoid working through the grief process. It is important to have the support of friends and family who will allow you your many mood swings and also give you the time and encouragement to face the reality of your loss.

c. PHYSICAL

Grief affects us physically. Some of the physical changes associated with grief are — lack of energy, tiredness, sleeping and eating problems, shortness of breath, weakness, weeping, crying, tightness in the chest and stomach. Studies on grief indicate that the immune system is disturbed during this traumatic stress causing our bodies to have less resistance to illnesses such as colds and pneumonia.

It is important to nurse yourself. You have a broken heart and it needs your attention to heal. You can be an active participant in your grief work. There are things you can do to feel better: drink lots of water, reduce your caffeine intake, reduce sugar consumption, eat foods with less fat, eat more fruit and vegetables, get at least 25 minutes exercise a day, rest even if you can't sleep, treat yourself gently.

APPENDIX 5
AIDS/HIV —
WHAT TO DO AS A CARE-GIVER*

If there is a single principle to keep in mind, it is: "It is up to the person living with AIDS/HIV to decide what kind of care they require." Sorting out when your help is needed and when it is not is something you will have to do by talking with your loved one and by listening to what they want. When faced with potentially fatal illness in someone they love, people tend to become overprotective, oversolicitous in trying to meet their loved one's every anticipated need. Relax. They will tell you what they need when they need it, if indeed anything at all. When in doubt, ask. And than respect the answer.

After receiving a positive HIV antibody test result, the first things your loved one will need from you are understanding, love, and respect. With no choice and frequently little warning, their life has been turned upside down and they are likely to feel very vulnerable, particularly for the first while. All they really need you to do at that point is to acknowledge their feelings and to stay with them as they come to terms with the reality of their life.

Once your loved one is past the initial shock, life may settle down for some time as the virus moves very slowly and years can pass before any symptoms become evident. Respect whatever decisions they make and offer whatever support you can as a friend. Try not to treat your loved one as a fragile invalid. People are still alive and thriving ten years after an HIV antibody positive diagnosis.

When illness does occur, let you loved one take the lead in deciding what to do. They may feel the need to get everything settled at once, from a living will to funeral arrangements. If this is their choice, then support it and help the process. But make sure you are doing this for their comfort, not yours or that of some other member of the family.

---

*Excerpted with kind permission of Persons with AIDS, Vancouver, B.C., 1994.

One of the most difficult decisions for your loved one will be whether to go into hospital or to stay at home in the face of serious illness. If homecare is to be a valid option, you must ensure that the level of care will be comprehensive and consistent. You do your loved one no favor by keeping them at home if they do not receive adequate care. By the same token, your loved one will probably need support and some advocacy to ensure that they receive personal attention in the hospital. Most hospitals welcome partners, close friends, and family.

Finally, take care of yourself and respect the fact that some of the care-giving will make difficult demands on you. Try to maintain a social life, see other friends, reach out for support when you need it. If you feel you need counselling, any of the AIDS organizations can refer you to a knowledgeable counselor.

APPENDIX 6
COGNITIVELY IMPAIRED AND HEAD INJURY*

a. COGNITIVELY IMPAIRED

Caregiving

Estimates indicate that millions of persons nationwide are caregivers; as many as 20-33% of families across the United States may be caring for an adult with a cognitive impairment. Cognitive impairments include a variety of diseases and disorders such as Alzheimer's disease, Parkinsons's disease, stroke, head injury, or AIDS dementia. Although each disorder has its own unique features, family members and caregivers often share common problems, situations and strategies, regardless of the diagnosis.

Cognitively impaired persons typically require special care, including (often 24-hour) supervision, specialized communication techniques, management of bizarre or difficult behaviors, incontinence, and help with activities of daily living (ADLs), e.g., bathing, eating, transferring from bed to a chair or wheelchair, toileting, and/or other personal care.

While each caregiving situation is different, caregivers are likely to experience enormous stress from their responsibilities in caring for a loved one. Many individuals become depressed or anxious and others report physical ailments associated with the stress of caregiving. For this reason, finding practical ways to cope and get help are especially important.

Brain-impaired individuals may experience a range of behavioral problems including communication difficulties, perseveration (fixation on/repetition of an idea or activity), aggressive or impulsive behaviors, lack of motivation, memory problems, incontinence, poor judgment and wandering.

---

*Excerpts from "Fact Sheet: Caregiving" by Family Caregiver Alliance, Bay Area Caregiver Resource Center, San Francisco, California.

b. HEAD INJURY STATISTICS

Head injury is a traumatic insult to the brain. Although not always visible, it may cause enduring physical, emotional, intellectual, and social changes for the survivor. The impact of head injury goes beyond the survivor. Long-term effects place an enormous emotional and financial burden on the individual's family, and strain medical and other service systems due to high costs and often life-long needs.

Magnitude of the problem

- Someone receives a head injury every 15 seconds in the United States. Every five minutes one of these individuals will die and another will become permanently disabled.

- Head injury is the leading cause of death and disability in children and young adults in the United States. It represents an estimated 13% of all injuries nationwide.

- Estimates for incidence of head injury vary. Researchers have generally concluded that head injury occurs in about 200 of every 100,000 people annually. Conservative estimates claim over two million individuals suffer a traumatic brain injury each year.

- About 500,000 to 750,000 head injuries each year are severe enough to require hospitalization; between 75,000-100,000 result in death.

Who is injured?

- Males are twice as likely as females to suffer head injuries.

- A head injury can strike at any age; however, head injuries disproportionately affect the young. Most survivors are between 15 to 24 years of age.

- Head injuries also affect the elderly at higher rates than the general population — about 211:100,000 for those age 75 and over.

Causes of head injury

- Motor vehicle accidents are the leading cause of head injuries — about 50%–60% in most studies. Falls are the second leading cause, followed by assaults and firearms.

- Motorcycle accidents claim responsibility for about 20% of transportation-related head injuries, about 12% are due to bicycle accidents.
- Alcohol plays a significant role in head injury accidents. About 56% of head injury survivors have a documentable blood alcohol level at the time of their accident.